Keto Body
The Ketogenic Diet, Bodybuilding and Tips for Rapid Fat Loss

This book includes:

(1) The Ketogenic Diet: *The Fast Way to Burning Fat*

(2) Bodybuilding: *How to Build the Body of a Greek God*

*** Tips for Rapid Fat Loss**

By Epic Rios

Intro

Thanks for purchasing *Keto Body: The Ketogenic Diet, Bodybuilding and Tips for Rapid Fat Loss.*

Before you begin reading *Keto Body,* make sure you take the time to read over the "Health and Fitness Chief Aim."

The "Health and Fitness Chief Aim" is a unique goal seeking tool designed to help you achieve your health and fitness goals.

Make sure to read over the instructions for the "Health and Fitness Chief Aim" and follow them correctly for creating your very own "Health and Fitness Chief Aim."

Thanks again for purchasing *Keto Body: The Ketogenic Diet, Bodybuilding and Tips for Rapid Fat Loss.*

I wish you great success with achieving your health and fitness goals.

Health and Fitness
Chief Aim

*Use the following guide for achieving your health and fitness goals.

Step #1

Write down your health and fitness goal(s) and be specific. For example, if you want to lose 10 pounds then write down, "I want to lose 10 pounds."

At the same time, if you want to build muscle, be specific and write down the amount of muscle you want to have. For example, if you want to have 10 pounds of muscle then write down, "I want to have 10 pounds of muscle."

Step #2

Write down the date by which you want to achieve your health and fitness goal(s).

For example, "I will lose 10 pounds by February 2019."

Example two, "I will be able to run 15 miles nonstop by May 2019."

Step 3

Write down what you are willing to sacrifice in order to achieve your health and fitness goals. In addition, write down what are you willing to give back (to the world) in return for achieving your health and fitness goal(s).

For example, "I am willing to give up drinking alcohol, specifically beer for the next 3 months in order to lose 20 pounds of fat. In addition, I am going to stop watching television after 10:00 PM and

I will instead go to sleep early so that I can wake up early and exercise."

"In return for achieving my health and fitness goals, I will serve as a role model inspiring and helping others to also achieve their health and fitness goals by sharing my knowledge, experience and wisdom."

Step 4
Repeat looking and reading over your Health and Fitness Chief Aim every day until you achieve your health and fitness goals. In addition, look and read over your Health and Fitness Chief Aim multiple times a day. Daily repetition is important for achieving any goal.

The Ketogenic Diet

The Fast Way to Burning Fat

By Epic Rios

"Pursue your health and fitness goals diligently, patiently and persistently and you are bound to be successful."   *– Epic Rios*

Table of Contents

There are no scenarios in which the publisher or the original author of this work can be in any fashion deemed liable for any hardship or damages that may befall them after undertaking information described herein.

Additionally, the information in the following pages is intended only for informational purposes and should thus be thought of as universal. As befitting its nature, it is presented without assurance regarding its prolonged validity or interim quality.

Trademarks that are mentioned are done without written consent and can in no way be considered an endorsement from the trademark holder.

Introduction

Congratulations on purchasing this book and thank you for doing so. The following chapters will discuss what you need to know to get started on the ketogenic diet.

This diet plan is one of the best diet plans out there because it is effective and it helps you to lose weight and burn off that stubborn fat that you have been working against for a long time.

Simply this effective book will provide you with all of the information that you need to fully understand and follow the ketogenic diet plan.

We will start out with some of the basics of the ketogenic diet, the benefits of this diet plan, how to eat properly, the best meal plans to help you get started, how the ketogenic diet and intermittent fasting can work together, and even how you can modify this diet plan for your workout plan.

Anyone is able to follow the ketogenic diet, and with the help of this educational book, you will be able to see amazing results with your fat and weight loss in no time.

When you have been trying other diet plans for some time and are not seeing the results that you would like, it may be time to change things up and try something new.

The ketogenic diet will effectively help you to see the results that you would like, and this resourceful book will give you all the information that you need to get started.

I want to take the time to thank you so much for choosing this book! Every effort was made to ensure it is full of as much useful information as possible, please enjoy!

Chapter 1: What is the Ketogenic Diet?

When you are ready to get started on a new diet plan, there are a lot of different options that you can choose from.

Some diets are going to be more like "fasting" where you need to cut out what you eat so much that it is very hard to stick with it.

Other diets will focus on cutting out all of the fats that you consume during the day so that you can focus on eating healthy carbs and lots of fruits and vegetables in your diet.

Some diets are healthy and some are not that healthy and there are often many people who swear by these healthy and unhealthy diets.

But think about this, which diet is actually going to give you the best results that you would like to practice when it comes to losing weight?

It is important to state that the ketogenic diet is one of the most effective diet plans that you can choose from.

The ketogenic diet plan is simple to understand.

In addition, learning and practicing the ketogenic diet is going to take away some of the common misconceptions about dieting, the misconceptions that have been holding you back from losing weight so that you can actually achieve your fat loss goals.

While many traditional diets, the ones that are considered really healthy, will ask you to eat more carbs and cut down on fats, the ketogenic diet takes things in a different direction.

With the ketogenic diet, you are going to severely limit the carbs that you take in and instead replace them with healthy fats that will increase your metabolism and make you feel amazing in no time.

The issue with normal diet plans is that you are taking in too many carbs. These carbs may seem healthy, but when the body breaks them down, they basically become sugars in the body.

If you are consuming additional foods that have sugars in them then this could add some additional issues to your health and prevent you from achieving your weight loss goals.

Keep this in mind - the body is used to consuming carbs for energy. So, the body is very happy when you take in some carbs and the body will use the carbs for energy.

The body will then transfer the carbs over to insulin and then try to use up the insulin. And when the body doesn't use up all of its insulin, then the body simply stores it as fat. As a result, a person will simply gain weight or not be able to lose fat as a result of the excess insulin.

Unfortunately, carbs are a very effective source of energy for most people. The body will often feel hungry and run down long before you use up the carbs that you consume, and you will eventually feel tired, grumpy, and hungry again.

This leads most people to eat more carbs in an effort to get their energy back.

After eating more carbs, people will feel better for a little while. But soon they will be tired and worn out again and the cycle just keeps going on and on.

Eventually you will end up eating way too many calories just to keep your energy levels up and all those extra carbs will be stored as excess body fat.

The ketogenic diet works to break this cycle. Instead of relying so much on eating carbs, you will instead rely on eating healthy fats.

You can still have some carbs, but the point is to push your body into **ketosis, a process where the body will use fats instead of carbs as its main source of energy**.

It is important to state that fat or "healthy fat" can be a really efficient source of energy.

While you will feel worn out and tired for the first few days as the body runs out of carbs (due to you eating fewer carbs), and starts looking for a new energy source, you will soon notice that your energy levels will start to go through the roof.

You will burn the "healthy fat" that you are eating as well as the "fats" that are stored in the body, all while feeling full and satisfied.

When you go on the ketogenic diet, you are responsible for cutting down the number of carbs that you consume.

On the ketogenic diet, most people will be limited to eating no more than fifty grams of carbs each day. In addition, most of these carbs will come from healthy sources like fruits and vegetables.

Some people like to push themselves into ketosis a little bit faster and will limit themselves to twenty grams of carbs a day or less.

However, it is advisable to slowly begin the ketogenic diet and to also slowly begin to reduce the number of carbs you eat each day.

Every person that practices the ketogenic diet needs to experiment with their carb intake based on their activity levels and other factors.

For example, people who do a lot of weightlifting, aerobics and cardio based exercises (swimming, running, etc.,) will need to take in slightly more carbs or above the fifty-gram recommendation to help them stay healthy and so that they can maintain being in ketosis.

(Ketosis is a process by which the body uses stored fat or body fat as fuel or energy. So, when very little carbs are consumed and that energy is used up, the body will go into ketosis in which the body will look to fat as an energy source for using as fuel or energy.)

Checking to see if you are in ketosis is very important if you are practicing the ketogenic diet.

You will only lose weight once you reach the state of ketosis and some people may need to adjust their food intake a bit more than others to see some weight loss results.

It is important to state that there are test strips available at pharmacies that you can buy that will allow you to check for the level of ketones in your body, so that you can adjust your diet early on and figure out what changes you need to make to your diet.

(Ketones are chemical substances that the body produces when there is not enough insulin produced in the body as a result of eating very few carbs.

So, the less carbs you eat the less insulin your body will produce resulting in ketones being produced by the body. So, ketones occur as a result of the body using fat as energy or fuel.)

Remember that when working with the ketogenic diet, you need to change up the way that you are eating on a regular basis.

You are not going to be able to eat a ton of bread and pasta and see results. However, lots of healthy oils and fats from healthy protein sources can help you to get the macronutrients that you need and to lose weight.

Carbs are not completely off limits, but you will be surprised at how quickly your daily allowance will disappear, especially if you are choosing bread and pasta as your carb sources.

Instead, you need to stick with healthy fruits and vegetables and learn how to go with the ones that are lower in carb content compared to others.

This makes it easier to get the vitamins and nutrients that your body needs without pushing the body out of ketosis.

Once you reach ketosis through healthy fats, moderate amounts of protein, and low carbs, you will need to maintain this diet for the long-term. As soon as you start to eat more carbs and go back to your old habits, you will get out of ketosis and can start to gain the weight again.

You can easily lose a lot of weight with the ketogenic diet, but you need to maintain the ketosis diet for the long-term if you really want to see the good results.

Following the ketogenic diet can be a bit difficult for some people. You may have to give up some of the foods that you have enjoyed in the past.

But once you learn a few of the rules that come with the ketogenic diet and you find a few favorite recipes that will help you to stay within the right macronutrient content for your body and for ketosis you are going to fall in love with the results.

The ketogenic diet may be hard in our modern world, but it is going to give you some amazing results with your weight and fat loss goals.

Understanding Ketosis

Ketosis is basically the process of your body relying on fats rather than on carbs or glucose to provide it with energy.

Most people eat enough carbs that they are going to rely on those for their source of energy. But this is not a very efficient form of energy.

You will quickly go through cycles of high energy and then crash when the carbs are all gone, and you will end up eating way more than you need just to keep your energy levels up.

With ketosis, you do not need to worry about your energy levels crashing and then trying to eat more carbs in order to increase your energy levels again.

Instead, you will teach the body to stop relying on carbs and instead the body will learn to rely on healthy fats that you start to take in.

When you eat healthy fats, ketones are going to be produced and used for energy.

Ketones will replace the glucose, giving you plenty of healthy energy without having to worry about the horrible crashes that glucose (sugars from carbs) causes.

Eating on the Ketogenic Diet

When you follow a ketogenic diet, you will consume at least 70 percent of your calories each day from fat.

The majority of the rest will come from protein, with only about five percent coming from healthy sources of carbs, such as low-carb vegetables.

As a beginner, you will need to build your meals around healthy sources of fats. These can include oils, cheese, nuts, meats, and fatty fish.

You can then add in some healthy sources of protein if they are not included already, as well as healthy low-carb options like vegetables and some fruits.

One thing to keep in mind on this diet plan is that you still need to take in moderate amounts of protein.

Many people get so focused on the fat intake and limiting their carbs that they forget to take in enough protein.

Protein is important to help you stay full and for preserving your body's muscles as well as keeping your muscles strong.

Negative Effects of This Diet Plan

You may also wonder if there are any negative effects of following this diet plan. Plain and simple, you are taking a large food group (carbs) and cutting it down to almost nothing on this diet plan.

For the most part, as soon as your body has time to adapt to ketosis, there shouldn't be any negative effects that you need to deal with.

You may feel a bit tired in the beginning as your body adapts, but once that adaption happens, you will find that you have more energy than ever before.

You should make sure that you have a wide variety of food options when it comes to eating on the ketogenic diet plan.

If you eat the same meals each day, or the same vegetables, you are going to miss out on important nutrients and this can cause some negative effects.

This is true of any diet plan if you do not add in variety. Make sure that you get plenty of variety in the diet, and you will see amazing results without any negative side effects.

Do I Need to Measure Ketones?

Many people choose to monitor the ketones that they consume. Actually, it is important that you monitor your ketones in order to ensure that you reach ketosis and that you stay within it to see weight loss results.

It is not necessarily a requirement for the diet plan, but it certainly helps. Measuring your ketones does not have to be difficult.

There are some testing strips that you can use that will tell you when you have entered ketosis and you can bring these out any time that you are worried about whether you are in the right range with your carbs or not.

Who Uses the Ketogenic Diet?

The biggest reason that people will choose to go on the ketogenic diet is to simply lose weight.

When you start relying on fat for your source of energy rather than glucose (sugars), you can melt off the weight and fat in no time.

However, there are many other reasons that people may choose to practice the ketogenic diet.

Originally, the ketogenic diet was designed to help patients who were dealing with a variety of neurological conditions, especially epilepsy.

It was found that young children who relied on a ketogenic-like diet were able to reduce the frequency of their seizures and reduce their medications.

Believe it or not, but there are some athletes who like to use the ketogenic diet to help with their endurance.

According to a paper that was released in the European Journal of Clinical Nutrition, there are a few other reasons that someone may choose to use the ketogenic diet.

These include:

- Evidence that the ketogenic diet can help people with high cholesterol, type 2 diabetes, weight loss, and epilepsy.

- New evidence has shown how the ketogenic diet may be able to help with a variety of neurological diseases like brain trauma, narcolepsy, Alzheimer's, and Parkinson's Disease, to name a few.

- People that suffer from cancer, severe acne, and even polycystic ovarian syndrome are often helped with the ketogenic diet as well.

Basically, anyone is able to use the ketogenic diet, whether they want to lose weight or are working to avoid one of the conditions named above.

The ketogenic diet is easy to follow and gives such amazing benefits to those who are able to follow it.

Chapter 2: The Benefits of the Ketogenic Diet

There are a lot of reasons that people will choose to use and practice the ketogenic diet. Simply, the ketogenic diet is one of the most effective diet plans out there.

In addition, the ketogenic diet can help resolve a variety of health issues that people are dealing with and not just with weight loss.

Some of the great benefits that you will receive when you decide to use and practice the ketogenic diet are:

- **Lose weight:** The number one reason that people choose to use the ketogenic diet is that they want to lose weight. And this diet plan is very effective at helping this to happen.

  Once your body enters into the process of ketosis and starts relying on fats for energy rather than carbs, you will see the weight melt off in no time.

- **Next, the ketogenic diet can help reduce cancer:** Some studies have shown how the ketogenic diet may be effective at reducing your risks of developing cancer.

  Cancer cells thrive when given lots of carbs, so if you take these carbs away, they will basically starve out. Regular healthy cells can rely on healthy fats for their nutrition, but cancer cells can't.

- **Next, the ketogenic diet will give you more energy:** During the first few days on the ketogenic diet, you may notice that you are feeling tired and worn down. This is because the body is so used to relying on carbs to stay energetic.

When you take those carbs away, the body is not sure where to find its energy source and may feel run down.

You just need to give it a few days, though; the body will start using the fats that you provide it for energy in no time. Once that happens, you will have more energy than ever before.

- **Next, the ketogenic diet will help lower your risk of diabetes:** With all those carbs you traditionally eat, it is common to see a risk of diabetes.

   You have to be very careful of the carbs you eat because the body will treat some carbs you eat just like sugars once they are eaten and broken down.

   So, if you are eating some sugars and lots of carbs, you are raising your insulin levels and increasing the amount of risk you have for diabetes.

   Cut out a lot of those carbs, as well as the sugars, and your body can clean itself up and cut down on your risk of diabetes.

- **Next, the ketogenic diet will lower your blood pressure:** Many people who have gone on the ketogenic diet report that their blood pressures went down.

   Many of the foods that you consume on a regular diet will have a ton of sodium inside, which can raise your blood pressure.

   Add in all the processed foods, high amount of carbs, and even the bad fats, and it is no wonder that most people have bad high blood pressure.

The ketogenic diet cuts out a lot of these bad unhealthy foods out of your diet so that you can recover and get that blood pressure back to normal.

- **Next, the ketogenic diet is great for the heart:** The ketogenic diet can even help out with the health of your heart.

  The healthy fats that you consume will help to strengthen your heart. The healthy fats also deliver some of those healthy vitamins and nutrients over to the heart better than carbs do.

  So, once you are reducing some of the carbs, the ones that turn into sugars in the body, you are giving the heart a fighting chance to be healthy and strong again.

- **Next, the ketogenic diet clears the mind:** When you are able to cut down on the number of carbs that you consume, and the number of calories that you are consuming, you will find that your mind feels much clearer.

  It will feel amazing to remember things, to think things through critically, and to no longer have to deal with the brain fog that you may have suffered from before as a result of eating so many carbs.

- **Next, the ketogenic diet can help fight epilepsy:** Originally, the ketogenic diet was developed as a way to help children who were suffering from chronic epilepsy.

  The high fat and low carb ketogenic diet were effective at helping young children fight off epilepsy and kept the episodes away.

The ketogenic diet needed to be used over the long-term, usually for two years or more, but helped children to not have to deal with the horrible effects of their seizures and helped them to reduce the amount of medication they needed to take.

Almost everyone is able to benefit from the use of the ketogenic diet.

It is different compared to some of the other diet plans that are available on the market, but this is part of what makes it so successful compared to the other diet plans.

When you are ready to start losing weight and improving many other aspects of your health, then make sure to try out the ketogenic diet to help you out.

Chapter 3: The Side Effects of the Ketogenic Diet

Before you get started with the ketogenic diet, it is important to know that there are some side effects or using and practicing the ketogenic diet.

These side effects are not horrible side effects like what you may be used to with common medications, but it is still a good idea to know what to expect when you are getting started on this new diet plan.

Some of the side effects that you may encounter when you are on the ketogenic diet are:

Dizziness or Headaches

One of the first side effects that you may experience when you get started with the ketogenic diet includes dizziness and headaches.

Dizziness and headaches are really prevalent in those individuals who for a very long time consumed a lot of caffeine and sugar before starting the ketogenic diet.

Both caffeine and sugar are highly addictive and if you go cold turkey on them, you may have a few side effects during the beginning process of the ketogenic diet.

You may introduce a little caffeine or sugar later on in the ketogenic diet plan if you want, but for those individuals who experience having a lot of trouble starting this diet plan or who really are addicted to caffeine and sugar, it is best to cut them out completely.

The good news is that the symptoms of withdrawal are only going to last for a few days and they really are not that severe.

You may feel a little anxious or upset because you will crave the caffeine and sugars that you are trying to eliminate from your diet.

However, if you are able to overcome your cravings for caffeine and sugar during the initial process of the ketogenic diet, you will break the addictions and you will not feel so reliant on consuming them as much.

One thing that you may decide to try is to slowly cut out your sugar and caffeine intake before you go on the ketogenic diet.

This will help you to not have to deal with these withdrawal symptoms as much. This can make things easier since you will already be dealing with feeling tired as your body gets used to the fats instead of the carbs.

If you are thinking about going on the ketogenic diet, consider cutting down on the sugars and caffeine for at least a few weeks ahead of time and you will not have to deal with the headaches or the dizziness as much when you begin.

Leg Cramps

Some of those who decide to go on the ketogenic diet will complain of dealing with leg cramps, especially when they are trying to go to bed at night.

This is common when you are in the early phase of the ketogenic diet.

This is a big problem for those users who are not paying attention to their micronutrients on this diet plan and who are not taking in enough potassium on this diet plan.

There are a few things that you are able to do to make sure you are getting enough potassium.

You can first work to try and eat plenty of foods with healthy amounts of potassium in them.

If you are having trouble doing this, you may decide to take a supplement that has potassium inside of it.

Many beginners decide to take a potassium supplement to help prevent leg cramps because keeping track of the macronutrients and the micronutrients for good health can be difficult.

However, you need to work towards not depending on supplements and instead eat real foods that will provide you with all the nutrients your body needs without taking any supplements.

Constipation

If you are not watching your micronutrients when you are on the ketogenic diet, you may deal with the issue of constipation.

This can be really uncomfortable for most people to deal with and can make sticking with the ketogenic diet a bit difficult.

However, the solution to this problem is pretty simple.

To ensure that you are not going to deal with constipation on the ketogenic diet plan, make sure that the majority of carbs that you decide to eat come from healthy green vegetables, which are full of fiber.

You also need to drink a lot of water on this diet plan because water has been shown to combat and prevent constipation.

For those individuals who maybe are already dealing with constipation, you may try a laxative to help you out.

Bad Breath

Another side effect that you may need to deal with on the ketogenic diet is bad breath.

While on the ketogenic diet plan, the body is going to burn up fat so that you can use this fat as energy.

This is the process of ketosis and will help you to burn through fat in your diet and the fat that is sitting around your body.

Unfortunately, the ketones (burning fat used as energy) that are released in this process will leave you with bad breath and make your urine smell bad.

The smell is going to be a little bit different than you may experience when after eating smelly food or by those individuals who suffer from halitosis (bad breath resulting from health problems).

Some people even compare it to a fruity candy smell instead, but if you do not want your breath to smell at all, then it is important to find a few ways to get rid of the bad breath.

Chewing on some gum without sugar, using mouthwash, or chewing on parsley or mint can help to get rid of this smell while keeping you on the ketogenic diet.

Feeling Tired

There are many people who will get started on the ketogenic diet who claim they feel tired.

They get going on this plan and are excited about all the big promises of more energy when they eat more healthy fats and fewer carbs.

Then they start on this diet and the first few days or in the first week they will begin to feel really tired almost like they just don't have enough energy to get things done.

This is completely normal on the ketogenic diet and it is important to know that these energy lacking feelings are going to fade away pretty soon.

The reason that you feel so tired when you start the ketogenic diet is that the body basically doesn't have any fuel for energy.

Sure, you are taking in healthy foods and providing it with fuel, but the body is used to relying on carbs and doesn't know what it should do when you take the majority of those carbs away.

So, the body is basically searching around hoping that you will eat and take in the carbs that it needs for easy energy access.

When you don't eat carbs or consume enough carbs your body is basically working on very little to no energy for a little while.

The good news is that feeling tired is not going to last for a very long time. For most people, it takes less than a week for the body to start recognizing the fat as a good source of energy and it will switch over.

Once the body starts to realize that it can use fat for energy instead of carbs, you will start to notice a big change.

Your energy will come back in a big way and you will feel amazing in no time.

You will be able to keep going all day long, even with fewer calories, and will ensure that you feel great about this diet plan.

As you can see, none of these side effects are life-threatening or that big of a deal when it comes to the ketogenic diet.

These side effects can make you a little bit uncomfortable and may not be the most pleasant when you are dealing with bad breath and feeling tired.

However, these side effects will usually not last for a long time and once your body adjusts to the ketogenic diet plan, you will not have to worry about them any longer.

Chapter 4: Who Can Safely Go on the Ketogenic Diet?

In most cases, following the ketogenic diet is a great experience. There are so many great health benefits that you will be able to enjoy when it comes to the ketogenic diet.

Many people choose to go on the ketogenic diet because they are tired of not being able to lose weight or fight off all that excess fat that has been hanging around their body for a long time.

But weight loss is not the only reason that you may choose to go on the ketogenic diet. If you have been fighting diabetes and its side effects for some time, reducing the number of carbs and the glucose it produces can help combat this health issue.

If you are worried about your high cholesterol levels and high blood pressure, simply practicing and following the ketogenic diet plan can help you to reduce your risks with these health issues as well.

Even younger children who have been dealing with epilepsy and those children with other neurological conditions may be able to benefit with the help of the ketogenic diet.

The children may be able to reduce some of the symptoms that they are dealing with and some have even been able to no longer need to use the medication they are on when they accurately follow the ketogenic diet plan.

Anyone who is dealing with health diseases or wants to lose weight or just simply wants to live a healthier lifestyle will be able to discover that the ketogenic diet is a good tool to help them out.

It doesn't matter if you are a man or a woman, the ketogenic diet is the right option to help anyone.

Who Shouldn't Use the Ketogenic Diet?

There are so many people who are able to use the ketogenic diet. The ketogenic diet has a lot of benefits and it can help you to lose weight, fight off many health concerns, and help you to feel amazing in no time.

However, there are certain groups of people who should avoid and not practice the ketogenic diet.

Practicing the ketogenic diet plan can be detrimental to the health of some people and even make them feel sick.

Some of those individuals who should avoid the ketogenic diet are:

- Children and teenagers
- Women who are pregnant and breastfeeding
- Women with irregular menstrual cycles
- People that have issues with their thyroid glands
- People that suffer from adrenal fatigue
- High-level athletes who need carbs to help them function better

These groups of people will often not do as well with the ketogenic diet.

This is because they need special dietary requirements that are eliminated from their diet when they follow the ketogenic diet.

For example, a pregnant or nursing mother needs to take in carbs to help her baby to grow and eliminating these completely can result in a nutrient deficiency for the baby.

Teenagers and children often need some of the glucose that is found in carbs, or they need higher carb content from fruits and vegetables than the ketogenic diet allows.

This does not mean that these groups of people can't take some advice from the ketogenic diet to help them stay healthy.

For example, teenagers or pregnant women may choose to limit their carbs a bit, but not to the fifty grams a day that is recommended by the ketogenic diet.

Instead, teenagers or pregnant women can instead stick to eating healthy carbs like fruits and vegetables while reducing their intake of unhealthy carbs like the bread and pastas that they normally eat.

Teenagers or pregnant women can also consider increasing their healthy fat intake and eating good amounts of protein each day.

So basically, some of these groups of people can follow some of the principles of the ketogenic diet without following or practicing so many of the restrictions the actual diet requires.

If you fall into one of the groups above, it may be a good idea to talk to your doctor before attempting to go on this diet plan.

This will help you to determine if you really need the ketogenic diet and if it is actually a healthy option for you, especially if you are in one of the groups above.

Chapter 5: The Ketogenic Diet and Exercise

It is important to understand how exercise and your fitness performance can be affected by the ketogenic diet.

It is also important to understand that maybe your exercise routine/plan/goals may need to be changed a little bit as a result of practicing the ketogenic diet.

However, you will still see some great results from your fitness workouts while practicing the ketogenic diet.

In additional, habitual exercise combined with the ketogenic diet will help you to lose weight and fat faster than ever.

You may also need to add a few extra carbs to your diet in order to have the right amount of energy for achieving your health and fitness goals.

With the ketogenic diet, you are greatly reducing the number of carbs that you are consuming and since many athletes require carbs to help them stay energetic, you may be curious to know how this is going to affect your body when you enter ketosis.

You will need to keep a few things in mind when you get started on the ketogenic diet when it comes to exercising, but it is just fine to exercise on this diet and all the health benefits definitely make it worth your time.

First, we need to understand that the traditional view on weight loss, the idea that you just need to eat less and exercise for a longer period of time (while getting plenty of cardio in as well) is advice that is outdated and just won't work with the ketogenic diet.

To really lose weight and get that leaner frame that you have been looking for, the foods that you eat while on the ketogenic diet are what matter the most.

Eating recommended foods on the ketogenic diet like meats, seafood, and dairy are great ways to begin the ketogenic diet.

The most important thing you can do for weight loss and maintaining your energy levels is to pay attention to how well and how disciplined you are to following the ketogenic diet.

If you are able to remain in a steady state of ketosis, rather than coming in and out of it because you can't keep your carbs steady or low, you will see some amazing results.

Before you decide to start doing more and more of your regular physical exercise activities while on the ketogenic diet, make sure that you understand when your body is in ketosis as well as spend some time testing your ketone levels.

However, once you get used to how the ketogenic diet works, adding in exercise can provide you with a lot of good benefits to your health.

Physical exercise like strength training and lifting weights will help to make your bones stronger as well as build muscle and make you have that lean look you want.

In addition, physical exercise like strength training and lifting weights is also great for the heart.

And as long as you are taking in nutrients properly on the ketogenic diet, physical exercise can easily fit in with your new diet plan.

Just remember that when you are exercising while on the ketogenic diet, make sure to stay healthy, make sure your energy levels are good and don't harm yourself while practicing the ketogenic diet.

Why Should I Exercise on the Ketogenic Diet?

After learning a bit more about ketosis and how the body needs higher levels of carbs in order to properly perform the activities that you would like, you may think that ketosis is not the best for long-term exercise.

However, exercising while on the ketogenic diet actually provides the user with many benefits including:

- In one study, ultra-endurance athletes were asked to do a three-hour run.

  Those who ate a low carb diet for about twenty months on average had up to three times the fat burn compared to the athletes who followed a high-carb diet.

  Both of these groups were able to replenish the same amount of muscle glycogen when done.

- Studies have shown that ketosis can help to prevent fatigue in people who exercise for long periods of time.

  For example, people that strength train for 1 or 2 hours or people who do cardio exercise activities such as running have sufficient energy to complete their long workouts.

- Ketosis is great for helping to maintain your blood glucose levels, whether you are considered obese or not.

- With the help of keto-adaption (which we will talk about later on), low-carb ketogenic dieters are actually better able to perform various activities, even while taking in fewer carbs over time.

- You receive all the regular benefits of exercise. In addition to the benefits listed above, those individuals who are on the ketogenic diet are able to receive all the same benefits that they would receive on any other diet while working out.

  However, the main difference between the ketogenic diet and other diets is that the ketogenic diet uses fat as energy instead of carbs.

  Keep this in mind, exercising while on the ketogenic diet will help you to be in a better mood, lose weight, see fat loss, control your blood sugar levels, reduce blood pressure, and so much more.

  Everyone should consider starting on their own workout program and combining it with the ketogenic diet.

  It is important to state that having a good mixture of different exercises, from flexibility to strength training and some lower-intensity aerobics or cardio exercises, will help you to make the whole body strong and will prevent injuries along the way.

While you may need to take a little bit of time off from working out when you first get started with the ketogenic diet to help you adjust, most people are able to successfully work out while practicing the ketogenic diet.

By making a few adjustments to your ketogenic lifestyle and by watching how many carbs you eat as well as when you consume your carbs will make all the difference in the results that you see when it comes to achieving your weight loss goals.

Types of Exercises to do While on the Ketogenic Diet

Your nutritional needs are going to vary based on the exercise or exercises that you want to perform. But generally, you will be able to divide up exercises into four group.

These four groups of exercises include stability training, flexibility training, anaerobic exercises, and aerobic exercises.

Let's take a look at how each of these can work with the ketogenic diet:

- **Aerobic exercise:** Aerobic exercise is typically known as cardio (swimming, running, cycling) and it will be any activity that gets the heart up and running for more than three minutes.

  As a result, your body may require more carbs while practicing the ketogenic diet.

  If you do cardio exercises that are steady-state and lower in intensity like walking you are going to be concentrating on fat burning, which makes it a great exercise for the ketogenic diet.

- **Anaerobic exercise:** This type of exercise is going to have short bursts of energy throughout an exercise session, such as HIIT, powerlifting or explosive exercises.

  If you plan to do anaerobic exercises, you may need to take in more carbs because anaerobic exercises require a lot more carbs as their primary fuel source.

Make sure that when you combine anaerobic exercises with the ketogenic diet that you consume just a little more carbs just for the sake of making sure you have the necessary energy to complete your physical workouts.

- **Flexibility training:** It is a good idea to add some flexibility exercises to your fitness routine.

Flexibility training can be helpful for stretching out the muscles, improving your range of motion, and supporting the joints.

Flexibility training is often used to help prevent injuries from some of the other workouts that you may do.

Some examples of flexibility training are Yoga and just simple stretching exercises.

Flexibility training does not require a lot of carbs. As a result, the ketogenic diet is perfect for people that do Yoga or simple stretching exercises.

- **Stability exercises:** Stability exercises are exercises that work on your core or abdominal (abs) muscles as well as help improve your balance.

Stability exercises are good for helping control your body's movements, strengthen the muscles in the body, and can even improve your body's alignment.

Stability exercises do not require a lot of carbs.

As a result, the ketogenic diet is perfect for people that practice stability exercises.

Keep this in mind when you are exercising while practicing the ketogenic diet:

"Mix up your workouts as much as possible. Do a combination of all four types of exercises and or training mentioned above for the purpose of developing the type of body that you want.

At the same time always monitor your energy levels to make sure you are consuming just enough carbs while practicing the ketogenic diet.

If at any moment you are feeling too tired to complete your workout routine simply stop exercising, monitor your energy levels and see if you need to increase your carbs intake. Safety first."

It is important to state that as you practice the ketogenic diet and you reach ketosis, the intensity of your exercise workouts is going to matter quite a bit.

When you do low-intensity workouts like walking or Yoga, the body will rely more on fat as its energy source, so these workouts are the best for those on the ketogenic diet.

The high-intensity aerobic exercises, like jogging and running, and anaerobic exercises, like powerlifting and sprinting, are going to rely more on carbs as an energy source and are not the best exercises to do while practicing the ketogenic diet.

Just keep in mind that if you are going to do high-intensity exercises you may need to add some more carbs to your diet.

Picking a Targeted Ketogenic Diet (Variations)

So far, we have just been talking about the basic ketogenic diet. This is a great diet if you are looking to get started and you don't plan to do really intense workouts.

The ketogenic diet will often work for regular exercise and for a little bit of low-intensity activities as well.

But if you are planning on doing activities that are more intense, or you plan to exercise or workout more than three days out of the week to help with weight and fat loss, then it is time to consider a targeted ketogenic diet variation.

A targeted ketogenic diet variation will help you to adjust your diet so that you get enough carbs to help you achieve your fitness goals as well as keep you in ketosis.

Those higher intensity workouts, like lots of weightlifting and sprinting are not going to do well with the regular ketogenic diet so having a targeted ketogenic diet variation will help you get the results that you would like.

These targeted ketogenic diet variations will allow you to have some more carbs during the day so that you can maintain your activity levels.

This does not mean that you can go out and enjoy as many sodas and baked goods as you like.

You still need to get your carbs from keto approved foods, like fruits and vegetables, but you are allowed to increase your healthy carb intake.

A good thing to remember is that you should eat about 15 to 30 grams of fast acting carbs (which includes options like fruit) about twenty minutes before and after your workout.

This helps your muscles to get the glycogen that they need to do well during training and so that your muscles can recover.

Eating during that time period will ensure that the carbs are used for the workout, so you won't leave ketosis at all.

Options or Variations of the Ketogenic Diet

There are a few options for the ketogenic diet that you can pick based on the amount of physical activity that you plan to do.

The different ketogenic diet variations that you can choose from include:

- **The standard ketogenic diet:** With this diet option you will keep your total carb count between 20 to 50 grams each day.

- **The targeted ketogenic diet:** With this diet option, you will stick with the 20 to 50 grams of carbs each day. But you will plan out when you eat these carbs.

  You will want to get the majority, if not all, of these carbs about an hour or less before you do your exercise. This is the best option for athletes who like to do high-intensity activities like weightlifting, sprinting, CrossFit, etc.,

- **The cyclical ketogenic diet:** For this one, you will cut your carbs down to almost nothing for a few days.

  And then on the days that you want to do a higher-intensity workout, you will eat higher-carbs on that day. This should even out for the right amount of carbs throughout the week.

Depending on the exercises that you are doing you may find that the carb content is too low, and you are not taking in enough carbs to keep up with your activity levels.

If you want to know if you are in a state of ketosis, you can simply purchase some test strips at the local pharmacy that will help you to know whether you are in ketosis or not.

You may also be able to increase your carb intake a little bit and still remain in the state of ketosis.

However, it is important to be careful when you slightly increase your carbs intake because it is really easy to jump out of ketosis.

In addition, if you do jump out of ketosis then you will lose the benefits of the ketogenic diet plan if you aren't closely monitoring how many carbs you consume.

The good news is that most people are able to adapt to eating lower-carb diets and using fat to help them get the fuel that they need.

This may take a few weeks and you may not be as strong for those first few weeks as the body adjusts. However, the longer you remain on the ketogenic diet, the more the body can adapt to this diet plan.

After practicing the ketogenic diet for a while, your body will become more efficient at burning the fat and using up the ketones that are in the body.

With enough physical exercise and after a while of being on the ketogenic diet, you will be able to see some amazing results with your body as well as achieve whatever fitness goals you plan to achieve.

Chapter 6: What Should I Eat on the Ketogenic Diet?

One question that a lot of people will ask when getting started on the ketogenic diet is what they are allowed to eat.

Working with the right macronutrients is one of the most important parts of the ketogenic diet. You must make sure that you are eating plenty of healthy fats and low carbs so that you can stay in ketosis.

Actually, eating plenty of healthy fats and low carbs is going to be one of the most important things that you concentrate on when it comes to the ketogenic diet.

However, as long as the foods that you eat fit into these macronutrients, and you are getting plenty of vitamins and minerals from the fruits and vegetables you choose to eat, you will lose weight.

Before we look at the specific foods that you are able to eat on the ketogenic diet let's take a look at the macronutrients.

This is really important and will ensure that you are eating enough fats to stay energetic as well as keeping the carbs low enough so that you don't kick yourself out of ketosis.

Also, don't forget that it is important to eat healthy sources of protein rich foods so that you can keep your muscles big and strong.

First, let's take a look at the fats that you need to eat. It is recommended that you get somewhere between 70 to 75 percent of your daily calories from healthy fats.

You must make sure that these are healthy fats. Going to the local fast food restaurant and eating a big burger and fries will not count because these are bad fats that will not help out with the ketogenic diet.

Instead, eating healthy fats like olive oil, fats from dairy products, and fats that come in healthy protein sources are much better options.

You will also need to eat moderate amounts of protein as well. You will need between 15 and 20 percent of your daily calories from protein.

This helps to keep the muscles as strong as possible and can be especially important if you are someone who likes to work out a lot and wants to build muscle with the ketogenic diet plan. Stick with options like healthy fish, chicken, turkey, and ground beef.

And finally, most people will want to keep their carb intake down to five percent or lower. If you are really into weight lifting, you can sometimes go up to ten percent.

But, before you increase your carbs intake, make sure that you experiment and see if you are really in ketosis with the higher amount of carbs or not.

Remember, when choosing carbs to eat stick with healthy options like fruits and vegetables that will help to keep you feeling full.

In addition, eating healthy carbs like fruits and vegetables will give your body the vitamins and nutrients that your body needs.

If you are able to stick with these macronutrients, you will see great results with the ketogenic diet.

It will take some time to get used to which foods will fit into this diet plan, but once you get used to it, losing weight and fat will be easier than ever before.

Foods to Eat on the Ketogenic Diet

Sticking with the macronutrients that we talked about above is one of the most important things that you can do on this diet plan.

But putting this into a meal plan can be difficult when you first get started.

Some of the foods that you are able to enjoy when following the ketogenic diet include:

- **Meat:** There are many different types of meat that you can enjoy, and this will provide you with the protein and some of the fats that you need.

You can choose from options like fish, lamb, veal, pork, venison, chicken, quail, duck, and shellfish.

With chicken, make sure that you leave the skin on to help increase the fat content, but do not bread or batter any poultry that you eat.

Make sure that you do not eat any processed meats, though. If choosing canned fish options, make sure that the preservation method does not use any added sugar.

- **Eggs:** Many meals on the ketogenic diet will require you to eat eggs for the purpose of consuming both protein and healthy fat.

Because eggs have lots of healthy protein and fats, they can be eaten for breakfast, lunch or dinner.

- **Cheese:** For the most part, cheese is a good food to eat while on the ketogenic diet. There are a few carbs found in the different varieties of cheese, so make sure to read the labels carefully and then count the carbs before you eat them.

Some cheese may push you over your daily required carbs intake so make sure you keep track of other carbs you have eaten that day.

- **Vegetables:** Vegetables will contain most of the carbs that you are going to eat but try to keep this to a minimum.

  You should go with the green and leafy options because these are lower in carbs so options like lettuce, cabbage, kale, and watercress are great.

  You can also go with options like bean sprouts, cucumber, celery, broccoli, and asparagus.

- **Fruits:** You can enjoy some fruits on the ketogenic diet, but you need to be careful about which ones you eat.

  Some fruits can be higher in carbs compared to some of the other food options on the list and if you eat too many fruits, you will end up going over your daily required carbs intake.

  If you choose to add some fruits to your diet, carefully watch your portions and avoid going over on the carb content.

  One recommended fruit is the avocado. The avocado is a good source of healthy fat so try to make the avocado part of your ketogenic diet meal plan.

- **Nuts:** Nuts are a good source of healthy fats and protein so they are fine to eat as long as you eat them in moderation as a type of dessert or as a snack. Some recommended nuts are walnuts.

- **Cream, butter, and oils** are usually fine because they provide you with some healthy sources of fat.

- **Dry spices** and **fresh herbs** are great for the ketogenic diet. Dry spices and fresh herbs will help you to get some flavoring in your meals without adding in any extra carbs.

As you can see, while you do need to be careful with the macronutrients that you are consuming on the ketogenic diet, there are still some options that you can go with to eat great meals.

Mix and match some of the options that were mentioned above, and you will get tasty meals that are easy to make and will help you to lose weight without feeling hungry.

Foods to Avoid on the Ketogenic Diet

For the most part, if the foods are not listed in the section above, you should not consume them on the ketogenic diet.

Consuming foods that are not recommended for the ketogenic diet can add in too many bad fats, bad carbs, and sugars than your body does not need.

In addition, consuming foods that are not recommended for the ketogenic diet may kick you out of your ketosis state.

Keep in mind that you do not want to work hard to get into ketosis and then end up cheating yourself and getting kicked out of ketosis because you consumed foods that are not recommended for the ketogenic diet.

Some of the foods that you will need to avoid on the ketogenic diet are:

- **Bread and pasta:** Bread and pasta may seem healthy, but just a small serving can put you over your required daily carb intake.

  There are healthier alternatives, such as keto bread or using vegetables to make noodles, so you can still enjoy some of your favorite meals without having to worry about eating too many carbs.

- **Baked goods:** In between the excess carbs and sugars that are inside most baked goods, it is no wonder that baked goods are not allowed on the ketogenic diet.

  It is best to stick with eating a piece of fruit (especially if you can find one that is lower in carbs) for your snack rather than eating any of the baked goods that are available.

- **Processed frozen foods/meals:** Anything that you can find in the freezer section of your grocery store should be avoided.

  These may seem healthy, but the preservatives and carbs are extremely high and will kick you out of ketosis.

  It is best to just leave everything that is in the freezer section alone and stick with fresh and whole foods instead.

- **Sodas:** Some people choose to drink diet sodas when they are on the ketogenic and diet sodas are allowed. However, you should avoid regular sodas because of all the sugar that is inside of them.

- **Fast foods:** While you are on the ketogenic diet, you need to avoid going out to eat.

Fast foods are full of way too many carbs and bad fats and will instantly take you out of ketosis without much effort. Avoid fast foods and just cook your meals at home instead.

- **Deli meats:** Deli meats may seem like a good option to get your protein, but in reality, they are mostly processed and full of lots of carbs.

  It is best to avoid deli meats as much as possible and focus your time and energy on eating healthier proteins and carbs.

It is important that you eat the right foods when it comes to the ketogenic diet.

There are some other diet plans that will allow you to cheat on occasion, but when you cheat on the ketogenic diet, you lose all of your weight loss benefits.

If you would like to stay in ketosis and really lose weight, then make sure to avoid the foods mentioned above and you will see great results with the ketogenic diet.

Chapter 7: Simple Meal Plans for the Ketogenic Diet

One of the hardest things that many beginners have trouble with is figuring out what they need to eat on the ketogenic diet.

While they may understand how the macronutrients are supposed to work on the diet, they are worried about how to plan out their meals and how to make it work well for them.

Coming up with ideas for your ketogenic meal plans is one of the best things that you can do because it outlines what you need to eat for the whole week or longer if you like.

Now, we are going to look at a simple one-week meal plan that you can follow to get started on the ketogenic diet and see amazing results in no time.

Monday
Breakfast: Scrambled Eggs
Lunch: Keto Asian Salad
Dinner: Pesto Chicken Casserole

Tuesday
Breakfast: Cheese Roll-ups
Lunch: Egg Omelet
Dinner: Meat Pie

Wednesday
Breakfast: Frittata with Spinach
Lunch: Chicken Soup (No Noodle)
Dinner: Carbonara

Thursday
Breakfast: Dairy Free Latte
Lunch: Avocado and Goat Cheese Salad

Dinner: Keto Pizza

Friday
Breakfast: Mushroom Omelet
Lunch: Smoked Salmon
Dinner: Keto Tacos

Saturday
Breakfast: Baked Bacon Omelet
Lunch: Keto Quesadillas
Dinner: Asian Stir-Fry

Sunday
Breakfast: Berry Pancakes
Lunch: Italian Keto Plate
Dinner: Pork Chops

Keto Recipes

Recipe #1
Scrambled Eggs with Spinach
What's in it?
- Some salt
- Pepper
- Butter (1 oz.)
- Eggs (2)
- Spinach

How's it done?
Whisk together the eggs while adding the pepper and salt.

Add some butter to a skillet and let it warm up. When the butter is hot, pour the eggs and let them cook.

After two minutes, the eggs should be creamy. Add some spinach to your eggs and you can finish scrambling and enjoy!

Keto Recipe #2
Pesto Chicken Casserole
What's in it?
- Peppers
- Some salt
- Chopped garlic cloves (1)
- Diced feta cheese (8 oz.)
- Pitted olives (8 Tbsp.)
- Heavy whip cream (1.5 cups)
- Green pesto (3 oz.)
- Butter (2 oz.)
- Chicken thighs (1.5 lbs.)
- Leafy greens (5.3 oz.)
- Olive oil (4 Tbsp.)

How's it done?

1. Allow the oven to heat up to 400 degrees. While the oven is heating up, cut up the chicken thighs into pieces and season them with pepper and salt.

2. Add the chicken to a skillet and fry them with some butter to make them nice and brown.

3. In another bowl, mix together the heavy cream and the pesto. Place the chicken pieces into a prepared baking dish.

4. Top the chicken with the pesto, garlic, feta cheese, and olives. Place everything into the oven to bake.

5. After 30 minutes, the dish is done and ready to eat.

Keto Recipe #3
Cheese Roll-Ups
What's in it?
- Butter (2 oz.)
- Cheddar cheese (8 oz.)

How's it done?
1. Take the cheese slices onto a cutting board. Slice the butter with a cheese slicer so you end up with thin slices.

2. Cover each of these slices with some butter before rolling them up and then serve and eat.

Keto Recipe #4
Chicken Soup
What's in it?

- Sliced green cabbage (2 cups)
- Shredded chicken (1.5 lbs.)
- Carrot (1)
- Chicken broth (8 cups)
- Pepper (.25 tsp.)
- Salt (1 tsp.)
- Parsley (2 tsp.)
- Minced onion (2 Tbsp.)
- Garlic cloves (2)
- Mushrooms, sliced (6 oz.)
- Celery stalks (2)
- Butter (4 oz.)

How's it done?
1. Start this out by melting the butter in a pot. Slice up the mushrooms and the celery into small pieces.

2. Add these to a pot along with the garlic and dried onion and cook for a few minutes.

3. After this time, add the pepper, salt, parsley, carrot, and broth. Let it all simmer until they become tender.

4. Add the cabbage and the chicken and cook for about 12 more minutes so the noodles are tender before serving.

Keto Recipe #5
Keto Pizza
What's in it?
- *Crust*
- Shredded cheese (6 oz.)
- Eggs (4)
- *Toppings*
- Salt
- Pepper
- Olive oil (4 Tbsp.)
- Leafy greens (5.5 oz.)
- Olives
- Pepperoni (1.75 oz.)
- Shredded cheese (4.25 oz.)
- Dried oregano (1 tsp.)
- Tomato paste (3 Tbsp.)

How's it done?

1. Allow the oven to heat up to 400 degrees. While the oven warms up, take out a bowl and beat the cheese and eggs

together to make the crust. Spread this out on a prepared baking sheet, making one large pizza or two small pizzas.

2. Place the pizza(s) in the oven to bake. After 15 minutes, the crust will be golden and you can take the pizza(s) out of the oven.

3. Allow the temperature of your oven to get to 450 degrees. Spread out the tomato paste on your crust and add on the rest of the toppings.

4. Place the pizza(s) back into the oven for a bit and after ten minutes, the pizza(s) should be ready. Serve with some leafy green vegetables and enjoy.

Keto Recipe #6
Smoked Salmon
What's in it?
- Pepper
- Salt
- Lime (1/2)
- Olive oil (1 Tbsp.)
- Baby spinach (2 oz.)
- Mayo (1 cup)
- Smoked salmon (.75 lbs.)

How's it done?
1. To start, bring out a plate and put the lime wedge, spinach, salmon and some mayo all on one plate.

2. Drizzle a bit of oil on top of the spinach before seasoning with the pepper and the salt. Serve this right away and eat.

Keto Recipe #7

Mushroom Omelet
What's in it?
- Pepper
- Salt
- Mushrooms (3)
- Yellow onion (1/3)
- Shredded cheese (1 oz.)
- Butter (1 oz.)
- Eggs (3)

How's it done?
1. To start this recipe, bring out a mixing bowl and crack the eggs inside. Season the eggs with pepper and salt and continue whisking to make them frothy.

2. Melt some butter in a skillet and then when it is warm, add the egg mixture.

3. When you notice this omelet is firming but is still a bit raw, add the onion, mushrooms, and cheese to the top.

4. Use a spatula to ease around the edges of your omelet so you can fold it in half. Take off the heat and serve.

Keto Recipe #8
Keto Quesadillas
What's in it?
- *Tortillas*
- Salt (1/2 tsp.)
- Coconut flour (1 Tbsp.)
- Ground psyllium husk powder (1.5 tsp.)
- Cream cheese (6 oz.)
- Egg whites (2)
- Eggs (2)
- *Filling*

- Olive oil (1 Tbsp.)
- Leafy greens (1 oz.)
- Shredded cheese (5 oz.)

How's it done?
1. Allow the oven to heat up to 400 degrees. While the oven is heating up, beat together your egg whites and eggs for a few minutes to make them fluffy. Add the cream cheese to your eggs and mix until they are nice and smooth.

2. In another bowl, whisk together the coconut flour, psyllium husk powder, and salt. Next, add these ingredients to your bowl of eggs and cream cheese a little at a time.

3. When the batter is combined, let it sit for a bit so it becomes thick like pancake batter.

4. Place two baking sheets on the counter and add parchment paper. Pour three circles of the dough on each sheet and spread into thin rounds.

5. Next, place the two sheets of dough into the oven and let the dough cook for a bit. After five minutes, you can take the tortillas out.

6. When the tortillas have cooled down, place them onto a cutting board and add some cheese on the tortillas. Also, add

on some leafy green vegetables and the rest of the cheese on the tortilla and then top it with a second tortilla.

7. Take out a skillet and add in some oil. Fry each of the quesadillas in the skillet for a bit on each side, letting the cheese melt.

8. After this is done, cut up the quesadillas and then serve and eat.

Keto Recipe #9
Asian Stir-Fry
What's in it?
- Sesame oil (1 Tbsp.)
- Ginger (1 Tbsp.)
- Chili flakes (1 tsp)
- Sliced scallions (3)
- Garlic cloves (2)
- White wine vinegar (1 Tbsp.)
- Pepper (.25 tsp. or 1/4 tsp.)
- Onion powder (1 tsp.)
- Salt (1 tsp.)
- Ground beef (1.5 lbs.)
- Butter (5.5 oz.)
- Green cabbage (1.66 lbs.)
- *Wasabi Mayo*
- Wasabi paste (1 Tbsp.)
- Mayonnaise (1 cup)

How's it done?
1. Shred up the cabbage with your food processor. Add some butter to a frying pan and then fry your cabbage for a few minutes.

2. Add the vinegar and spices and cook for a few more minutes before putting the cabbage in a bowl.

3. Melt the remainder of the butter before adding the ginger, chili flakes, and garlic and then let it cook. Add the meat and let it get brown all the way through.

4. Add the cabbage and the scallions to this mixture and stir to make it hot. Top with sesame oil, pepper, and salt.

5. Before serving, mix the ingredients together with the mayonnaise. Serve this stir-fry with some of the wasabi mayo on top.

Keto Recipe #10
Keto Pancakes
What's in it?
- Butter (2 oz.)
- Ground psyllium husk powder (1 Tbsp.)
- Cottage cheese (7 oz.)
- Eggs (4)
- *Toppings Below*
- Whipping cream (1 cup)
- Fresh berries (8 Tbsp.)

How's it done?
1. To start this recipe, take out a bowl and blend all the batter ingredients together. Set the bowl to the side and let it expand for at least five minutes.

2. When you are ready, heat up a bit of the oil in a pan. Add some of the batter to the pan and let the batter cook for three

minutes on both sides. Make sure to flip the batter (pancake) carefully.

3. Turn off the heat when the pancake is done and serve with the heavy cream and the berries of your choice before enjoying your meal.

Chapter 8: The Ketogenic Diet vs. Intermittent Fasting

The ketogenic diet can be a very effective diet plan.

If you are able to eat the right foods and closely monitor your macronutrients, you will enter into ketosis and see big results.

Still, some people hit a rut with their weight loss goals or simply need to do even more to help improve their overall health.

As a result, working with just the ketogenic diet may not be enough for some people.   One diet alternative that people can choose to practice is called intermittent fasting.

What is Intermittent Fasting?

Intermittent fasting is more of a lifestyle than a diet. Intermittent fasting is simply fasting or not eating food for a certain period of time.

Now that period of time of fasting or not eating food is usually between 12-16 hours. However, many people experience better results by fasting for 16 or more hours.

There are a lot of different variations when it comes to intermittent fasting, so you can choose the method that works the best for your schedule or for you to maintain for the long term.

Let's take a look at some of the basics of intermittent fasting so you can see how it will work well with the ketogenic diet.

The Intermittent Fasting Approach

There are actually a few different approaches that you can use when it comes to intermittent fasting.

Each intermittent fasting approach can be effective, and it is often based on what
fits your schedule.

The most common approaches that you can use with intermittent fasting are:

- **Skipping meals:** With this option, you will skip over a meal or two so that you can induce some extra time for fasting.

  So, for example, skipping breakfast or simply not eating in the morning can be one intermittent fasting approach.

  Skipping breakfast is one of the most effective methods for practicing intermittent fasting simply because you are already fasting all night from you last meal (dinner).

  If you must eat breakfast every morning than maybe try to skip either lunch and simply eat dinner.

  The benefit of this intermittent fasting approach is that it allows you to experiment to see what works for you and your schedule.

- **Eating windows:** With this intermittent fasting approach, you are going to work on getting all of your macronutrients within a certain eating schedule.

  For example, a person can have an eating window from 12:00 PM-7:00 PM. So, this means a person can eat from 12:00 PM – 7:00 PM.

  So, while most people eat from when they get up until when they go to bed, a personal practicing this intermittent fasting approach will reduce their eating time to windows of four to eight hours depending on their work and lifestyle schedules.

For example, you can have an eating window from 8:00 AM – 4:00 PM. So, this means you can only eat between 8:00 AM – 4:00 PM.

So, within this eating window you can eat two or three small meals. This intermittent fasting approach is good because you can experiment to see what is convenient for your work and lifestyle schedules.

- **One to two-day cleanses:** With this intermittent fasting approach, you are going to put yourself on an extended fasting period.

  With one to two-day cleanses, you will simply avoid eating for one or two days. You can do one or two-day cleanses once or twice a week.

  Now this intermittent fasting approach will effectively reduce the number of calories that you consume resulting in great weight loss.

  Most people will find that it is hard to start out with a one or two day fast, which is why restricting your eating window or skipping meals are two of the best intermittent fasting approaches you can choose from.

  Remember to experiment with intermittent fasting and try out different eating windows for a week or so to see what intermittent fasting approach works best for you.

How Does Intermittent Fasting Work?

While there are a few different options when it comes to choosing an intermittent fasting approach, you may wonder why it can be so effective.

The whole point of intermittent fasting is to simply eat food during a certain period of time.

Our bodies will only be able to take in so much food at once, so if we are only allowed to eat for a few hours during the day and then fast during the rest, we are limiting our calorie intake which results in weight loss.

During the fasting time, we are not allowed to eat at all. Our metabolism also seems to speed up as long as the fasting period is short, such as fasting for just eighteen hours rather than for a whole week or more.

So not only are we reducing the calories that we are able to consume because our bodies can't take in that much food at one time, we are also speeding up our metabolism at the same time.

Over time, your body is going to learn how to adjust to intermittent fasting.

In the beginning, intermittent fasting is going to be hard and you may feel hungry during the fasting period.

But if you can maintain your periods of fasting, the body will eventually adapt and you will be able to feel just fine without eating all day long.

In addition, maintaining your periods of fasting and keeping track of the food you eat will eventually become easier when you only have a few hours a day to eat.

It is important to state that when you are in a fasting state, the body is able to break down some of the extra fat that is being stored by your body.

Now if you include ketosis from the ketogenic diet, all of the excess fat that you have on your body will simply melt off in no time.

In addition, you will still have plenty of energy for all of your daily activities.

Ketosis actually mimics the fasting state because we take the glucose out of our bloodstream so that we can use fats as our main source of energy.

During your fast, the body is going to rely on those extra fat stores to help you to stay energized.

If you are doing intermittent fasting along with the ketogenic diet, you need to make sure that you really get the sufficient amount of fat content that the body needs so that the body can get the right amounts of energy that it needs.

It is important to state that when you combine both intermittent fasting and the ketogenic diet together, you will be able to burn through fat, lower your glucose levels, and see tremendous results in your overall health.

Intermittent fasting is not necessarily for weight loss, although it can help you to lose weight if you are prone to overeating throughout the day.

In addition, intermittent fasting can help you reduce your calorie intake resulting in weight loss.

When you combine intermittent fasting with the ketogenic diet, you are sure to see some tremendous weight loss results as well as an increase in your health benefits.

Are the Ketogenic Diet and Intermittent Fasting Similar?

There are a few similarities that you will find with the ketogenic diet and intermittent fasting.

Both are going to work to limit the amount of glucose in your diet so that the body will start to rely more on using fats for energy rather than carbs and sugars for energy.

This is an effective way to melt the fat off your body and help you to lose weight.

However, the methods that both use to help you reach this result are different. The ketogenic diet helps you to use fat as energy by changing up the macronutrients that you consume to cut out the carbs.

Intermittent fasting will help you to burn fat because you will be forced to reduce how many calories you are able to consume as a result of having a small eating window.

The ketogenic diet is an eating plan. With the ketogenic diet you have certain foods that you are able to consume, and you need to stick with eating those specific foods if you want to be on this diet plan.

On the other hand, intermittent fasting can be done with any type of diet plan. However, intermittent fasting will not be effective if you only eat junk food during your eating window.

But you can combine intermittent fasting with other diets such as the Mediterranean diet, or any other diet plan that you choose.

But when intermittent fasting is combined with the ketogenic diet, you are going to get some amazing weight loss results and your overall health will greatly improve.

Can I Use Intermittent Fasting and the Ketogenic Diet Together?

Yes, it is possible to use both intermittent fasting and the ketogenic diet together.

Keep in mind, intermittent fasting is more about fasting or not eating for a certain period of time each and every day and that period of time can be between 12-16 hours or more.

Now the ketogenic diet is more about the types of foods that you would eat each and every day specifically low carbs, a lot of healthy fats and moderate protein.

It is important to state that you do not have to go on an intermittent fasting diet in order to lose weight with the ketogenic diet.

It is already hard enough for many people to follow the ketogenic diet so combining both intermittent fasting and the ketogenic diet for weight loss is not required, but instead an option.

But for those people who would like to experiment and seek to achieve their weight loss goals and improve their overall health, then combining both intermittent fasting and the ketogenic diet is definitely a great idea.

With intermittent fasting, you will limit the hours that you are able to eat. Instead of allowing yourself to spread your meals and your snacks all throughout the day, you will limit your "eating window" to just a few hours a day.

With intermittent fasting, many people will choose to only eat between 10:00 AM - 6:00 PM and eat all of their macronutrients during this time period.

Others will do a whole day of fasting once or twice a week where they are not allowed to eat at all for one full day.

When people do a full day of fasting they try to consume all of their nutrients on the other days of the week in order to have sufficient energy for their one full day of fasting.

Just keep in mind that the point of intermittent fasting is that you are limiting the amount of time that you are able to eat which forces you to eat fewer calories which results in weight loss.

Now if you ever feel like you hit a plateau with your weight loss goals while on the ketogenic diet, simply consider combining the ketogenic diet with intermittent fasting.

Combining both the ketogenic diet and intermittent fasting will definitely "shock" the body and you will also benefit greatly by burning more fat and achieving your weight loss goals.

When you combine intermittent fasting with the ketogenic diet, you must remember to stick with the macronutrients that we discussed above that are approved for the ketogenic diet.

So, you will still stick with a high fat, moderate protein, and low carb diet plan even while intermittent fasting.

You will just need to be more careful about the times you eat those macronutrients, but otherwise, you can follow the ketogenic diet exactly the same.

If you want to get some of the benefits that come with intermittent fasting or you want to increase your weight loss, then combining intermittent fasting with the ketogenic diet can be very effective.

You can experiment with the different types of intermittent fasting variations that are available to see which one fits into your schedule and works best for you.

Of course, if you find the ketogenic diet is effective enough or adding in intermittent fasting is too difficult, you can always just stay with the ketogenic diet on its own and still see some amazing results.

Conclusion

Thank you for making it through the end of this book.

I hope the book was educational, informative and able to provide you with all of the tools you need to achieve your health and weight loss goals or whatever they may be.

The next step is to get started with the ketogenic diet.

This is one of the most effective diet plans that is available for helping you to lose weight.

While you will need to get used to some of the dietary changes that are unusual compared to other traditional diet plans, the ketogenic diet will really help you to lose weight in no time.

So, what you have come to learn from this book is what exactly the ketogenic diet is all about and how you can use it for your own weight loss journey.

You have learned the basics of the ketogenic diet, the benefits of trying it out, how you can use it with intermittent fasting to lose more weight, the foods that are allowed on the ketogenic diet, and even some meal plans to help you get started.

It is important to mention that the more information that you have before starting the ketogenic diet, the more you will be successful with this diet.

Just keep in mind that when you are tired of trying out all the other diet plans that haven't been successful in the past and you want to work with something that will actually work, the ketogenic diet is always a great option for weight loss.

Thanks again for choosing to read my book and I wish you great success with the ketogenic diet.

67

Health and Fitness
Chief Aim

*Use the following guide for achieving your health and fitness goals.

Step 1
Write down your health and fitness goal(s) and be specific. For example, if you want to lose 10 pounds then write down, "I want to lose 10 pounds."

At the same time, if you want to build muscle, be specific and write down the amount of muscle you want to have. For example, if you want to have 10 pounds of muscle then write down, "I want to have 10 pounds of muscle."

Step 2
Write down the date by which you want to achieve your health and fitness goal(s).

For example, "I will lose 10 pounds by February 2019."

Example two, "I will be able to run 15 miles nonstop by May 2019."

Step 3
Write down what you are willing to sacrifice in order to achieve your health and fitness goals. In addition, write down what are you willing to give back (to the world) in return for achieving your health and fitness goal(s).

For example, "I am willing to give up drinking alcohol, specifically beer for the next 3 months in order to lose 20 pounds of fat. In addition, I am going to stop watching television after 10:00 PM and

I will instead go to sleep early so that I can wake up early and exercise."

"In return for achieving my health and fitness goals, I will serve as a role model inspiring and helping others to also achieve their health and fitness goals by sharing my knowledge, experience and wisdom."

Step 4

Repeat looking and reading over your Health and Fitness Chief Aim every day until you achieve your health and fitness goals. In addition, look and read over your Health and Fitness Chief Aim multiple times a day. Daily repetition is important for achieving any goal.

Bodybuilding

How to Build the Body of a Greek God

By Epic Rios

Table of Contents

There are no scenarios in which the publisher or the original author of this work can be in any fashion deemed liable for any hardship or damages that may befall them after undertaking information described herein.

Additionally, the information found on the following pages is intended for informational purposes only and should thus be considered, universal.

As befitting its nature, the information presented is without assurance regarding its continued validity or interim quality.

Trademarks that mentioned are done without written consent and can in no way be considered an endorsement from the trademark holder.

Introduction

Congratulations on purchasing your personal copy of *Bodybuilding: How to Build the Body of a Greek God.*

Thank you for doing so.

These days, bodybuilding information is everywhere.

Building muscular big bodies seems to be the norm, but is that really what you are looking for? And at what cost are you willing to build a big body?

This book looks at the classic Greek God physique, one that is strong and capable of achieving great things.

With big, clunky bodies becoming the norm for good physiques these days, it is important to have an alternative for people that don't want a big, overly muscular body.

It is important to state that the ancient Greek body is one that was built on hard work and military training.

In addition, the ancient Greeks did not focus on putting in long hours of weight training at the gym every day.

Instead, the ancient Greeks were hardworking warriors and farmers and their bodies reflected that functionality.

The following chapters will discuss how to create a modern-day workout with focus on the old Greek ways of bodybuilding in order to build a healthy, strong body that is more than just a showpiece.

This book will also discuss specific workouts and nutrition plans that will help you achieve your ideal body.

By reading this book, you will discover how important maintaining an overall healthy lifestyle is in creating an ideal Greek body.

In addition, you will also realize how your mental, physical and overall quality of life will greatly improve as a result of developing and maintaining your new physique.

It is important to state that there are plenty of books on bodybuilding on the market, but none are quite like this.

Thanks again for choosing to purchase this book. Also, every effort was made to ensure this book provides you with as much useful information as possible. Please enjoy!

Chapter 1: Greek Bodies in Art - Drawings and Statues

In order to truly understand what you are striving for with building a Greek physique, it is important to understand the history behind the ideal Greek body, as it is a rich and vibrant one.

First off, the Greek empire existed from 800 BC to 146 BC, about three thousand years ago.

Even though it was so long ago, ancient Greek culture is still influencing civilizations around the world, including the modern-day health and fitness culture.

A major theme in Greek art throughout the centuries has been to maintain good order and form.

The goal with any piece of art is to draw the eye and keep it by presenting something that makes sense to the eye and to the brain.

By using subjects that have perfect proportions, the human eye will constantly be drawn to looking at a figure, statue or piece of art.

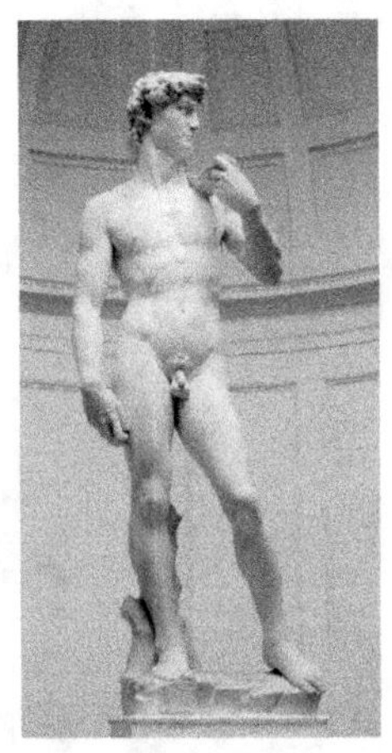

These concepts of subjects that have perfect proportions have been reflected in the work of well to do modern artists

When it comes to art and statues, the main focus for the ancient Greeks was to create a human form that was IDEAL and PLEASING to the human eye.

According to the ancient Greeks, the Greek body was considered an ideal standard to the ancient Greeks for a number of reasons.

One reason was that the ancient Greeks wanted to have the reputation of being a strong and conquering society portrayed by an ideal Greek body.

Although modern day Greece is very different today than what it used to be, the ancient Greek empire reached all the way to what is now considered the Middle East.

The ancient Greek citizens were considered some of the most fearsome warriors of their time and war was constantly glorified.

The ancient Greeks were very proud of their society and they expressed it through their art by creating Greek Gods with ideal eye-catching proportions.

The strong and pioneering Greek soldiers' body became a model as the ideal Greek.

What is interesting and often forgotten in modern society is that the ancient Greeks manufactured these ideal images in the likeness of Gods in which they have never actually met.

Just like in all religions, the idea of God is just that, an idea.

Although Gods are just figures in a person's imagination, the human mind simply creates an image that it finds appealing and this is something the ancient Greeks were very good at.

The ancient Greeks were very good at developing these ideal Gods that reflected their warrior like society and they were very proud of these ideal Gods.

Although the ancient Greeks creation of Gods and superhuman figures were not born out of reality but out of imagination, the Greeks believed it was their DUTY to uphold and live up to these imaginary images.

These days you will see superhuman figures created by artists using Photoshop that are not a true reflection of modern day society.

Just like the ancient Greeks, modern day society tries to live up to these ideal Photoshop images and people unsuccessfully fail to achieve the ideal body image they want to achieve because these ideal body images are not real.

Simply, many people dream of having a perfect body with perfect form but in nature and in reality, a perfect body doesn't exist.

Even people that have plastic surgery still do not have a perfect body because there will always be a flaw and an imperfection that can be pointed out and recognized.

It is important to state that an important event that made the ancient Greeks very popular was the creation of the Olympics.

When the ancient Greeks established the Olympics, they created games where they could display the strength and stamina of their people.

In addition, the Greeks believed that participating and succeeding at these Olympic games was an important time to display their more than ideal physiques.

While the focus was on winning at the Olympic games, it was a great opportunity for the ancient Greeks to display the beauty and power of their ideal bodies.

The first Olympics was held in honor of Zeus, the most respected of all the Greek Gods.

Interestingly, nudity was common at the Olympic games because the ancient Greeks believed that the human body was something of beauty and should be worshipped.

As a result, the ancient Greeks thought it would be a great idea for participants to display their nude artistic looking physiques during the Olympic games.

The belief system of ancient Greece also brought rise to the idealistic body.

In Greek mythology, a total of fourteen Gods existed, all of which had their own strengths.

Zeus, who was the most powerful of all the Greek Gods, was the God of Thunder and Sky.

There was also Hades, the God of the Underworld, and Apollo, the God of the Sun, among others.

What all the male Greek Gods had in common were their marvelous physiques.

Regardless of their power and personal strength, ancient Greek Gods were portrayed following a natural form that was most physically appealing to the human eye.

Ancient Greek art always depicted the Greeks Gods as perfect creatures, who existed in a form that was in great proportion.

Even today you can see paintings and sculptures that display well-proportioned athletic Greek bodies.

Some of the most famous artworks and sculptures were created during the classical period of Greece, between 500 and 300 B.C.

This period influenced the Roman Empire and had the most lasting impression through art and civilization surviving worldwide in modern times.

The classical period of Greece was also a time in which Greek artists did their best work to recreate the ideal human form thought to be a direct liking to the bodies of Greeks Gods.

During the classical period of Greece, the proper ratios of the human body were extensively studied.

The ancient Greeks were so obsessed with the ideal human form that they were one of the first civilizations to quantify proper ratios of waist to height, waist and shoulder width and other body proportions.

These important body ratios will be discussed in more detail in the next chapter.

Famous works of art like Discobolus, a statue of a Greek athlete throwing a discus, is a very iconic statue that shows a strong and powerful Greek body in action.

This sculpture shows the athletes agility and the body's range of motion as well as the development of muscle and brute strength required to be an ideal figure for the ancient Greeks.

It is important to remember that the Olympics originated in ancient Greece and the Greek athletes were the best of the best.

The ancient Greeks athletic bodies were hard and strong and the athletes were able to participate in all the games, including wresting, boxing and running events.

Another popular ancient Greek sculpture is "The David," created by Michelangelo during the Renaissance period.

This popular ancient Greek sculpture is a work of art that cannot be compared to any other.

"The David" depicts a young man of stellar form simply standing there, at about seventeen feet tall.

With a modest smile and oblivious attitude, this young man is simply in all his glory; a Greek man.

The musculature and details of "The David" show a man in his true, perfect form.

Speaking of Michelangelo, he was also responsible for creating beautiful works of art in the Sistine Chapel in Vatican City.

Michelangelo's painting on the ceiling of the Sistine Chapel in Vatican City called, "The Creation of Adam" is one of the most famous pieces of art ever created.

This famous piece of art shows an iconic image of when God first created Adam, the first human.

It shows the hands of God and Adam reaching out to each other to touch each other's hands.

It is important to state that the bodies of both Adam and God are shown in ideal proportions, typical of ancient Greek art.

In addition, you can clearly see the purity of both figures because they have been painted in a way that depicts flawless bodies; something to be attained.

Interestingly, the bodies of ancient Greek women and goddesses are idealized in a much different way than we see in modern times.

Modern day's standard of beauty says that women should be very thin yet display a bit of muscularity.

Looking at ancient Greek art, we cannot compare these modern standards to the influences from ancient Greece.

In fact, ancient Greek women were idolized for being slender but not "sickly" thin like modern day female "models."

Ancient Greek women were in proper proportion with their waists. They were slender but their hips were large and showed the ability to bear children.

Ancient Greek women were known to be healthy and it was very important in ancient Greece for women to have a healthy figure for bearing children.

In addition, there were no chiseled female chins or emphasis on rock hard abs like modern day female bodybuilders or women CrossFit warriors.

Instead, ancient Greece was a more lenient time for women, as womens primary role was to bear children and serve as a caregiver.

Similarly, the standard for the male physique, since ancient Greek times, has also changed as well.

For example, there was a major shift in the late twentieth century that morphed the ideal ancient Greek male figure into that of a superhero.

So late twentieth century male fitness figures would begin to have muscles that were required to be big and overdeveloped regardless of being functional.

In addition, late twentieth century male fitness figures would be bulky and their upper bodies were much larger than their lower bodies.

Think of modern day bodybuilders and men who use steroids to gain mass, yet lack function and athleticism.

Modern day overly developed muscular bodies are so far against the ideal, functional warrior body of the ancient Greek.

These days, we have traded function and athleticism for "gym and beach muscles," specifically the chest and arm muscles.

In addition, many modern-day bodybuilders can bench press 300 pounds but they don't have the functionality to carry a suitcase up the stairs or lack the conditioning to run 1 mile at an easy pace.

For the ancient Greeks, they took great pride in having the ability to use their ideal bodies to fight in wars, maintain their homes and provide food for their families.

It is important to state that the ancient Greeks did not have any modern-day tools or equipment to do any heavy lifting of objects or structures.

Instead, the ancient Greeks simply used brute strength and a strong willingness to move, function, complete any task and survive on a daily basis.

Chapter 2: Proportions of Greek Gods

Ancient Greeks took their physiques very seriously.

For the ancient Greeks, it was considered a sign of strength, power and strong character to maintain a certain physique.

This was modeled after the perfection of Greek Gods, who were considered immortal and strong by the ancient Greeks.

The ancient Greeks even went as far as to consider specific measurements of the human body to be desirable.

Much like bodybuilders today, the ancient Greeks were obsessed with obtaining a perfect body.

However, unlike modern day bodybuilders, the perfect Greek body was one that was functional, athletic and strong.

It is important to state that ancient Greece was often in war and it needed healthy, strong warriors to maintain their armies and fight their enemies.

As a result, the ancient Greeks trained as fearless warriors and it was deemed necessary to have a strong, functional body to even have a fighting chance against their enemies.

Ancient Greek men trained to be powerful, agile and fast in order to defeat their enemies.

Fearless Greek warriors were naturally lean, carrying very little body fat. They also had strong upper bodies but did not have overly developed chest and arm muscles like current day bodybuilders.

It was important for ancient Greek warriors to have great stamina in order to run and be able to travel on foot to new battle fields to fight against their enemies.

Stamina was a huge part of training for ancient Greek warriors.

Being able to run long distances to a battle field without getting tired and then upon arrival be ready to fight with NO REST was an absolute must for an ancient Greek warrior.

Those Greek warriors who did not have the stamina to keep up with the rest of the Greek warriors would be left behind and would be the first to die in battle.

For the ancient Greek warriors, they simply trained to survive and not just to look good naked.

These days, there are fewer opportunities to fight in battle. In addition, modern day armies have available vehicles and planes to move people around as well as sophisticated weaponry to prevent hand to hand combat.

As a result, there is no real reason for any modern day "soldier" to really train as a warrior when sophisticated technology can do all the fighting for them.

It is important to state that ancient Greek warriors were often in face-to-face combat with their enemies, using swords and shields as their weapons.

In addition, the Greek warriors were required to have tremendous strength and stamina in order to use their swords and shields effectively in battle without getting tired.

Even Greek men who were not part of the Greek military and did not fight in battle were considered strong, athletic and ready for battle if needed.

Those Greek men who were not fighting were farmers and workers who spent their days working in the fields, growing crops and responsible for the agriculture of ancient Greece.

These Greek men working in the fields were tough. They would work long days lifting crops and items over their heads while pulling on their livestock at the same time.

These Greek famers rarely were in situations in which they would need to bench press weights or perform barbell curls.

Instead, these Greek farmers had functional strength, the kind that is required for every day survival and that is required for getting real work done.

It is important to state that the ideal measurements of a strong working Greek man were as follows: for the bicep it was **16.4 inches in diameter**.

As compared to a modern bodybuilder, a strong working Greek man's bicep is considered small.

In addition, during the ancient Greek era, the ideal neck for a Greek man was **16.8 inches in diameter,** the ideal chest was **45.5-inches in diameter** and the ideal forearms were **13.2 inches in diameter.**

These ideal measurements seem like very specific body ratios to aim for but if you were a Greek man, reaching these goals was a matter of day to day survival and living.

As for the lower body ideal measurements for a Greek man, it is first important to state that the ancient Greeks had naturally strong and muscular legs.

In addition, ancient Greek men were required to be able to run long distances, be agile enough to evade enemies and strong enough to work as farmers and perform daily chores.

As a result, a Greek man was required to have legs that were functional and not overly muscular or bulky in order to remain functional for day to day living.

The lower body ideal measurements for a Greek man are as follows:

A perfect thigh was **24.1 inches in diameter** and the calf muscle was **15.5 inches in diameter.**

Now that you know a little about the ancient Greeks upper and lower body ideal measurements, let us now focus on the abdomen.

The ancient Greeks were known to have a very strong core.

As you may or may not know, the abdomen and back are the muscles at the center of every physical movement.

The abdomen allows for the arms and legs to swing in a controlled manner.

The ancient Greeks were known to have slim athletic bodies that were not overly built. In addition, their waists were in direction proportion to the rest of their bodies.

An ideal perfect waist for a Greek man was **31.9 inches in diameter** and an ideal perfect hip ratio was **38.7 inches in diameter.**

Hearing about the ancient Greeks perfect body measurements may seem like a bit of a turn-off.

In addition, you may ask yourself, "How on earth is an everyday person able to achieve such ideal body standards?"

Truthfully, it is very difficult to achieve the ancient Greeks ideal body standards because everyone's body type and bone structure is different.

However, once you know your body type, you can then work on developing a near perfect body like the ancient Greeks.

If you don't know what your body type is consider that there are three body types that most people are considered to fit into.

The three body types are:

1. Ectomorph

2. Mesomorph and

3. Endomorph

An **Ectomorph** is a person that is naturally thin and has a very thin bone structure.

In addition, an Ectomorph may have a hard time gaining weight and as a result a person with this body type remains naturally thin.

A **Mesomorph** is a person that has more of a "desired" body type because this person is neither thin nor big but instead this body type fits perfectly between an **Ectomorph** and an **Endomorph**.

An **Endomorph** is a person that has more of a "round shape" body type. In addition, the bone structure of this body type tends to be bigger and wider than the other body types.

Once you figure out which body type you may have, you can then work on creating a physique like the ancient Greeks according to your body type.

As you learn about the ancient Greeks ideal body measurements and their obsession with the human body, it is important to state that you should not get discouraged with achieving your health and fitness goals.

In all honestly, it will be very difficult to attain and maintain a body like the ancient Greeks believed a human body should look like so don't focus too much on these ideal body measurements.

Instead, consider the **Golden Ratio**, a term and a number that is much simpler to understand.

The Golden Ratio is a mathematical figure that was used during ancient Greece that many artists often believed expressed an ideal body displaying both beauty and balance.

As a result, the Golden Ratio was used to portray balance and beauty in many paintings and sculptures during the Renaissance period.

It is even said that Da Vinci himself used the Golden Ratio for defining all the proportions and dimensions for his paintings.

As you can see, the ideal body proportions of ancient Greek statues are a reflection of the Golden Ratio.

So rather than focusing on obtaining ideal body measurements according to the ancient Greeks, it is a lot more important to look at the overall proportions of your very own measurements.

However, modern research shows that when it comes to human attraction, men who fit a certain "ideal body ratio" are considered scientifically more attractive to women.

For example, the ancient Greek male physique was known to have broad shoulders with a narrow waist and hips that produced a "V-shaped" look.

And even in modern times, research shows that men that display a "V-shaped" look are considered more attractive by women.

What can also be said about the ideal body measurements of the ancient Greeks was that they believed it was very important for the neck, arms and calves to all have the same measurements in order to contribute to the ideal Greek body type.

The ancient Greeks believed so strongly that their perception of ideal body measurements were very attractive and pleasing to the human eye and so that is why they regarded them so highly.

It can be said that the same way the Golden Ratio was used to expressed an ideal body during ancient Greek times, the human face also follows a similar ratio.

For example, research shows that ideal facial features should be symmetrical and aligned in a way that follows a natural order.

In addition, faces that are symmetrical and aligned well are considered the most attractive.

To develop a body that is ideal to your proportions consider that your waist circumference should be 40-50% of your height.

So, if you are six feet tall, or 72 inches tall, your ideal waist size is between 28 and 36 inches.

Knowing your ideal waist size can help you determine your ideal shoulder size as well.

If you exercise and you truly want to make sure your overall body is well proportioned without being overly muscular or bulky, simply consider your lower body to be well proportioned to your upper body.

So, you don't want to have an overdeveloped upper body and an underdeveloped lower body.

Instead, you want to train to make sure your upper and lower body are well proportioned to each other.

You also want to consider that your calves should measure about the same as your biceps and your thighs should be strong yet slender.

Sometimes people are naturally born with big calves and legs but this does not mean that your arms and biceps should be equally as big.

Naturally, the human body can only get so muscular without steroids.

So, if you are looking to develop a naturally looking, well-proportioned body like the ancient Greeks, then aim for developing a body that is more "athletic" looking vs a bodybuilder's physique.

To put things in perspective, the ideal Greek body was described as one with broad shoulders, strong and without overly developed arms.

In addition, the chest was required to be strong, tapering down to a slim, yet muscular core. And the legs of an ideal Greek physique were required to be muscular but lean.

The ideal Greek physique was meant to be functional and ready for war and not meant to be shown off for vanity.

Nowadays, many men enjoy wearing tighter clothing that helps them show off their physiques and that is simply because they are trying to attract women or impress people.

Keep in mind that in clothes, a modern day Greek body looks slender but toned. In addition, there should be no bulging muscles trying to escape your t-shirt.

Remember that we all have certain features about ourselves that we cannot change.

Things dictated by our genetics like the shape of our faces or the proportions of our bone structures cannot be changed unless you are considering plastic surgery.

What you can do is use good nutrition and total body workouts to develop toned muscles and reduce your body fat percentage.

If you want to develop a body like the ancient Greeks then use the ideal ancient Greek physique as a benchmark in order to guide yourself with the proper nutrition and training that is required.

It is important to state that obtaining a near perfect body like the ancient Greeks may be very difficult to achieve.

Instead, focus on improving your health and fitness levels and enjoy yourself along the process.

Chapter 3: How Hollywood Portrays Greek Gods

Although a lot of things have changed since ancient Greece, our physical bodies and body types have not.

In addition, it is still very possible to achieve a body like the ancient Greeks but it does require a lot of hard work and commitment.

Just take Hollywood actors for example.

There are many Hollywood actors that have been able to achieve a body similar to the ancient Greeks and this has been clearly portrayed in movies.

Hollywood actors have even gone so far as to develop bodies that are strong and functional similar to the ancient Greeks.

Remember, the ancient Greeks were required to have a strong body yet its primary purpose was to be "functional."

If you look at famous Hollywood actor Brad Pitt, he was able to transform himself into a Godlike warrior known as "Achilles" in the movie "Troy."

In the movie "Troy," "Achilles" is known for being a fierce warrior that displayed great strength and agility.

If you analyze Brad Pitt's physique in the movie "Troy," you do not see him with bulging bodybuilder type of muscles.

Instead, his muscles are toned and he is very athletic displaying tremendous speed, power and agility.

In addition, Brad Pitt's midsection is long and lean with strong, well-chiseled arms and legs.

Although the physiques of Hollywood actors may not always seem to be realistic, what can be said is that with proper nutrition, training and exercise, an average looking person can most certainly transform themselves to look like a modern day athletic Greek warrior.

Another Brad Pitt movie that has become a "classic" among men as a result of his godlike body is the 1999 movie "Fight Club."

In the movie "Fight Club," Brad Pitt plays the role of "Tyler Durden," the founding member of an underground fight club where members of the group fight each other bare knuckled and without rules.

Although the role that Brad Pitt plays in the movie "Fight Club" is very different then the role he played in the movie "Troy," he is still able to display an amazing godlike physique in the movie "Fight Club."

For example, in the movie "Fight Club," Brad Pitt has a very long but lean, athletic body almost displaying more of a "boxer's" physique.

In addition, Brad Pitt appears to be very "cut" and able to display very defined 6-pack abs in the movie "Fight Club."

"Tyler Durden," as Brad Pitt is referred to in the movie "Fight Club" is meant to look scrappy, squirrely and a little bit crazy.

In addition, Brad Pitt's face is chiseled as a result of having very little body fat and his muscles are well defined.

Overall, Brad Pitt's body in the movie "Fight Club" is designed to show that it is meant for fighting and destroying others.

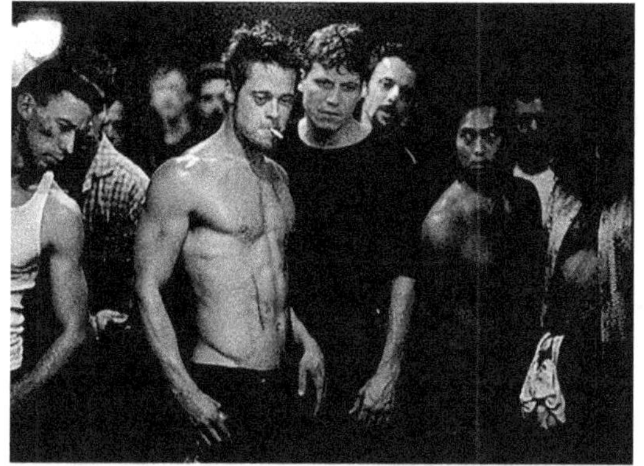

There are many fascinating movies that show ancient warriors with godlike physiques like the movie "Troy" and the very popular "300" which is about the famous 300 Spartans.

However, in the past few years, Superhero movies have become quite popular with many people as a result of the action in the movies and the muscular physiques of the Superheroes.

It is important to state that there is a great distinction between the ancient Greek God body and the Superhero body.

While the ancient Greek God body and the Superhero body are both strong and muscular, the Superhero body is very similar to the body of a modern-day bodybuilder.

It is important to state that the art of Bodybuilding slowly became more and more popular in the 1940s.

In addition, there was a massive push by the bodybuilders to display just how big their muscles can get.

Bodybuilders, since the 1940's have focused on developing extremely large upper bodies while maintaining very tiny waists.

In addition, the idea of having proper Greek proportions was totally disregarded and forgotten by bodybuilders.

Bodybuilders also focused on pure aesthetics disregarding developing a "functional" physique which was the result of hard work by the ancient Greeks.

Bodybuilding competitions also quickly took off in the 1940's with top contenders having very large, sometimes steroid induced chest and bicep muscles with tiny, almost womanlike waists.

Bodybuilders later began to use tanning products and baby oil during bodybuilding competitions for the purpose of enhancing muscle definition.

Back in the days of the ancient Greeks, there was no need for using tanning products and baby oil for the purpose of displaying a well-defined physique.

Instead, the ancient Greeks developed an aesthetically warriorlike physique as a result of every day hard work and survival.

While a bit exaggerated, the Superhero body, which can be currently seen in several movies, has adopted more of a bodybuilder's physique then the ancient Greek God warrior physique.

This is because every year we see more and more people pushing their bodies to get bigger and bigger with the help of steroids and performance enhancing drugs.

As a result, having a big bulky body has become the norm in the fitness and entertainment industries including Hollywood's portrayal of Superheroes and their bodybuilder type physiques in movies like Captain America and Thor.

These days, Marvel Comics and other comic book giants have made movies of just about every Superhero out there.

Popular Superheroes like Superman and Thor are displayed on covers of DVDs all over the world. Their upper bodies are large and in charge, almost carrying too much muscle to be of any real help.

Chris Hemsworth, the actor that plays Thor in the most recent Avengers series has a typical modern day overly muscular superhero build.

While his muscles and physique are something to be admired, the look of his body is very different from the ideal ancient Greek warrior physique.

Even today, cartoon depictions of superheroes are even more exaggerated than ever.

Take a look at the character "Metroman" in the Dreamworks movie "Megamind."

"Metroman" has a huge upper body and a very small waist and very thin legs.

Yes, "Metroman" is just a cartoon character but this overly muscular cartoon Superhero reinforces the idea that having a large upper body is the new standard of strength when it comes to Superheroes even if it is just a cartoon.

Chapter 4: Build Muscle Like a Greek God

Getting the body of a Greek God may actually be easier and more productive than you think.

Remember that ancient Greek ideal bodies were that of functional human beings. So, this means that the ancient Greeks did NOT have ideal bodies for the mere purpose of showing off their muscles.

Instead, the ancient Greeks were proud of their physiques as a result of training hard every day as warriors ready for battle.

In addition, the ancient Greeks also worked very hard in the fields growing crops to feed their families.

As you can see, the ancient Greeks were able to build muscle by doing physical labor and not by counting endless repetitions in a weight room.

Now in order to develop a workout routine that will help you develop a physique like the ancient Greek warriors, it is important to first consider exactly what the ancient Greeks did to develop their physiques.

In addition, it is also important to consider how to go about naturally transforming your body whether at home or at a gym.

There are currently many fitness companies and gyms that exist that purposely (or not) design exercise routines that build strength through functional exercise.

Perhaps the most popular right now is CrossFit.

Another popular fitness organization that helps fitness enthusiasts to build strength through functional exercise is the Ultimate Fighting Championship or (UFC).

Although you may not have the desire to be a UFC fighter, training in mixed martial arts is an excellent way for developing a warriorlike physique similar to the ancient Greeks.

So, in order to develop a body like the ancient Greeks you have to consider what kinds of functional exercises are required to develop a warriorlike physique.

Some good functional exercises are bodyweight exercises such as:

1. Pull-ups
2. Parallel bar dips
3. Pushups
4. Bodyweight squats
5. Jumping squats
6. Lunges
7. Jumping lunges

Some good functional exercises using fitness equipment can be:

1. Medicine ball exercises such as medicine ball throws
2. Kettlebell exercises such as kettlebell walks or "farmer walks"
3. Dumbbell exercises such as dumbbell squats to shoulder press

4. Jump rope exercises such as explosive jump roping with "double unders" and "criss-crosses"

Remember that the ancient Greeks did not rely on heavy equipment for getting in shape. Instead, they would run, wrestle, box and use brute strength to move large objects.

However, modern day gyms provide a wide variety of training equipment for getting in shape and it is just a matter of learning how to use the equipment for developing a functional body.

It is important to state that the ancient Greeks placed great emphasis on cardio and having the conditioning to run far distances without getting tired was very important to the ancient Greeks.

Some great cardio exercises that would greatly improve your conditioning are:

1. Circuit training using dumbbells, medicine balls, bodyweight exercises or machines
2. Stair running or Running Sprints
3. Using an Indoor Rowing Machine
4. Jump Roping or Skipping Rope
5. Mixed Martials Arts – Specifically Boxing, Muay Thai or Wrestling
6. Plyometric Exercises like jumping squats and burpees

As you can see, a combination of functional strength training exercises combined with effective cardio exercises would make you very athletic and functional.

In addition, a combination of both strength training and cardio type of exercises will most definitely help you develop a physique like the ancient Greeks.

While we will discuss cardio in more detail in the next chapter, just remember that it needs to be integrated into your training routines for developing a lean, functional physique.

That being said, a fitness trend that has become very popular in the fitness world is High Intensity Interval Training or HIIT for short.

High Intensity Interval Training, or HIIT combines small bursts of intense cardio activity usually between 20-90 seconds followed by some rest.

What makes High Intensity Interval Training so popular with many fitness enthusiasts is that it burns fat and can even build muscle in a short amount of time.

You can even do bodyweight exercises and use kettlebells, medicine balls or dumbbells for getting a good high intensity interval training workout.

When it comes to developing a modern-day warrior body like the ancient Greeks it is important to consider what muscles to exercise in order to get the best and fastest results.

Something to keep in mind is that the three largest muscles of the human body are the **legs, back and chest muscles.**

So, when you exercise you want to make sure you focus on exercising these three large muscle groups.

To develop a well-rounded functional body like the ancient Greeks, it is important to consider doing **total body strength training exercises** that work the three largest muscles in the body.

In addition, making effective cardio workouts part of your fitness training will greatly improve your results of achieving a well-rounded functional body like the ancient Greeks.

It is important to state that traditional bodybuilding focuses too much on getting big muscles and displaying overly developed bodies that serve no real-world purpose.

As a result, if you truly want to develop a physique like the ancient Greeks then it is important to train your body to be a lean, functional athletic machine that is ready for anything.

Here are some sample workouts routines that you can use to get you started with your fitness training:

<u>Bodyweight Routine I</u>

1. Chin-ups (5-8 repetitions)

2. Pushups (8-10 repetitions)

3. Lunges (12-15 repetitions)

Rest for 30-40 seconds and repeat for 5 sets

Perform each exercise one after the other with no rest

<u>Circuit Training Routine II</u>

1. Dumbbell Goblet squats (10-15 repetitions)

2. Dumbbell rows (8-12 repetitions)

3. Dumbbell bench press (8-12 repetitions)

4. Dumbbell lunges (10-15 repetitions)

5. 30 second plank (abs) exercise

Rest for 30-40 seconds and repeat for 5 sets

Perform each exercise one after the other with no rest

Strength and Plyometric Training Routine III

1.   "farmer walks" using dumbbells or kettlebells

2.   Jump rope for 1 minute

Rest for 30-40 seconds and repeat for 5 sets

As you can see from the three sample training routines, these methods of training are very different compared to bodybuilding routines.

While the ancient Greeks had their methods of training for getting fit, it is important for you to develop your own methods, routines and training for developing your own physique.

Remember, the key to a Greek body is training that requires moderate weight for strength training for the purpose of building firm and functional muscles.

Keep in mind that making the goal to lift as much weight as humanly possible will get you more of a superhero type of body instead of a Greek warrior body.

Always keep the goal in mind to build functional strength without overdoing it.

The good news is, you don't need to spend countless hours at the gym to get a great body.

Instead, you just need to train in a manner that keeps you lean and fit.

In addition, seek to always be "evolving" with your training in order to remain motivated with achieving your health and fitness goals.

Another thing to consider is that weight training in the gym no longer means you have to be doing the so called, "best exercises" for getting fit.

Instead, think about the fitness goals you want to achieve. Next, develop a plan to achieve your fitness goals. Finally, take action for achieving your fitness goals.

So, if your fitness goals are to develop a body like a Greek warrior, then train in a functional manner that will produce those results.

In addition, don't fall into the trap of having to do certain or specific exercises for getting in shape.

Instead, experiment with a variety of exercises, fitness routines and training equipment for getting the best results when it comes to achieving your fitness goals.

Consider that the ancient Greeks did not perform exercises like the barbell squat or deadlift because squatting heavy weight and deadlifting did not serve them any purpose in battle or in everyday living.

Simply the bodies of the ancient Greeks were not built for squatting or deadlifting hundreds of pounds, repetition after repetition because for them it was unnecessary to do so.

Just looking at an ideal Greek figure, we can tell that the ancient Greeks were not bench pressing excessive weight, as their chests were defined but not huge like modern day bodybuilders.

While using weight machines and free weights can mimic functional exercise, it can only go so far.

This is why interval training and doing activities that combine muscle training with real life situations is so important.

Remember, interval training is a method of doing a combination of high intense exercise followed by low intense exercise.

For example, running sprints for 50 yards giving 100% effort followed by very light jogging giving 50% effort would be considered interval training.

As you can see by this example of interval training, this type of training would have been beneficial to the ancient Greeks especially during wartime.

Although in the beginning, there were no available gyms in ancient Greece for Greek warriors to train, Greek warriors simply trained outside in public view.

Eventually, training in public view led to establishments for training and learning which later became known as "Gymnasiums."

The ancient Greeks believed the human body was such a beautiful art form that they would even go so far as to exercise naked at Gymnasiums.

Something to keep in mind is that whenever ancient Greek warriors did train, they never counted repetitions.

Instead, the ancient Greeks trained to simply improve their fitness levels as well as for preparing themselves for warfare.

It is important to state that Greek warriors would practice fighting, boxing, wrestling and they practiced training to fight using their powerful swords.

Today, we can recreate some of this type of training with mixed martial arts training.

When it comes to developing a body like an ancient Greek warrior, consider focusing your time on taking classes that combine lots of disciplines and training that the ancient Greeks would likely be doing.

For example, you can seek to improve your flexibility by learning Yoga. You can also seek to improve your breathing and your ability to relax and concentrate by practicing meditation.

You can even expand on your athletic pursuits by learning new fitness skills like advanced calisthenics or learning how to swim like a pro.

The most important thing you must do for developing a body like an ancient Greek warrior is to simply take action.

In addition, develop a strong willingness for achieving your Greek warrior physique and don't make excuses.

What is great about this very moment is that we are living in a time where we have access to all kinds of fitness training, state of the art gyms and equipment.

In addition, there is an abundance of available information on nutrition, dieting and overall health.

Therefore, it is a lot easier NOW to build a functional physique than it was when the ancient Greeks did it.

It is important to state that there is no one specific way for developing a body like the ancient Greeks.

To build a functional and well-proportioned body like the ancient Greeks consider the following steps:

1) **Develop a plan for getting fit.** This includes the types of exercises you will do, the type of equipment you will use, how often you will exercise and for how long you will exercise for.

2) **Focus on your nutrition.** Nutrition is extremely important for developing a lean, functional physique like the ancient Greeks.

   Consider what foods you will be required to eat for getting lean and fit. We will discuss nutrition later in the following chapters.

3) **Make a commitment.** Make a commitment to yourself for taking the necessary action and following through with achieving the body you want to have.

   In addition, consider how you will transform your body and look in 3 months, 6 months, 9 months and in 1 year.

Following these steps will most definitely help you to build a functional and well-proportioned body like the ancient Greeks

As stated before, there is no one specific way for developing a body like the ancient Greeks.

Instead it is a matter of experimenting with different types of exercises, equipment, fitness routines and training.

Many people believe that going to a gym and lifting heavy weights is the only way for developing a lean, functional physique but this is not true.

Instead, consider that you can exercise at home using bodyweight exercises. You can also exercise outside running sprints.

You can even do a combination of running sprints and then perform bodyweight exercises like pushups while you rest.

It is important to use your creative mind for getting lean and developing a functional body.

When you use your creative mind for getting lean and fit, you develop a sense of curiosity for seeing what is possible.

In addition, you learn more about what you can achieve both physically and mentally when you use your creative mind for getting fit.

You also keep yourself motivated along your journey for developing and achieving the type of body you want to have.

Below are 3 very important areas you want to focus on when developing your Greek warrior physique:

1) **Strength** – Strength is important for having a strong body. However, lifting extremely heavy weight is not required for developing a lean, functional physique.

   Instead, simply focus on doing what is challenging for you and always keep safety in mind.

2) **Conditioning** - Conditioning is important because it allows you to develop endurance so that you will not get tired so easily and so that you can push through your workouts.

   In addition, it is not enough to simply develop a good-looking body. Instead, developing a functional body, a body that is useful, a body that does not get tired so easily is the goal behind developing a Greek warrior physique.

3) **Flexibility** – Flexibility is important because it prevents your body from getting very stiff and losing its range of motion.

   In addition, you will have more mobility and you will move better as a result of having more flexibility. You will also avoid injuries as a result of developing more flexibility throughout your body.

As you can see, focusing on developing strength, conditioning and flexibility will help you develop the physique of an ancient Greek warrior.

In addition, you will become lean, functional and athletic as a result of focusing on strength, conditioning and flexibly.

To give you an example of how one particular Greek God was able to develop his lean, functional body, let's look at Poseidon, the God of the Sea, Horses, Storms and Earthquakes.

Poseidon, was most notably known as God of the Sea and protector of all waters because of his excellent swimming abilities.

Poseidon had the ability to stay underwater for long periods of time.

In addition, Poseidon was also known as an "Olympian God" that participated in the ancient Greek Olympic Games.

Poseidon was strong, athletic and resembled Zeus, the God of Sky and Thunder.

Now some people may be thinking, "How can swimming help me develop the body of a Greek warrior?"

In addition, some people may consider swimming to be more of a cardio type of exercise instead of a strength training exercise. However, this is simply not true.

Swimming is a unique total body workout that can help you develop speed, balance, agility, coordination, strength and improve your overall athleticism.

Now you may be asking, "But what if I don't know how to swim?"

Consider that in the past ten years, more and more athletic coaches have been making swimming pool workouts part of their athletes training and recovery programs.

For example, aside from using a swimming pool to simply swim sprints and perform various swim strokes, you can actually run in a swimming pool both in the shallow and deep end.

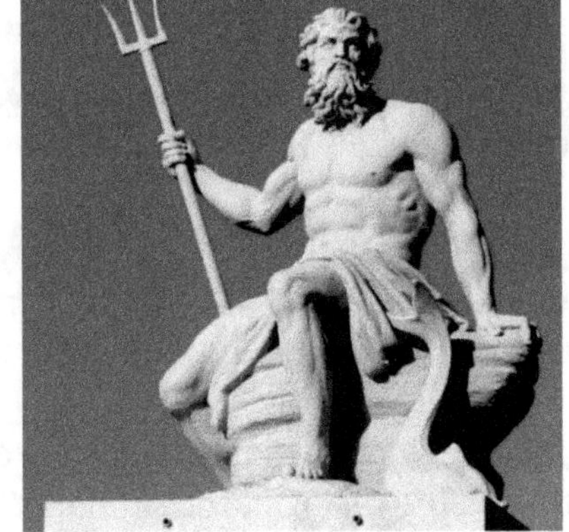

Poseidon, God of the Sea

You can also perform plyometric exercises in a swimming pool such as jumping squats, jumping lunges and tuck squats.

You can also do resistance training exercises in a swimming pool using your own bodyweight, specialized dumbbells and other training equipment.

As stated before, there is NO one specific way for developing a physique like the ancient Greeks.

Therefore, it is important to keep an open mind, experiment with various exercises, training and workouts and stay committed to achieving your health and fitness goals.

Chapter 5: Cutting Fat with Cardio

Getting lean, fit and developing a functional body is what is required for developing a physique like the ancient Greeks.

However, for many people getting extremely lean is very difficult to do especially in modern times because of easy access to all kinds of unhealthy foods.

Keep in mind that when you exercise you will develop some muscle. But unless you focus on developing a lean body, then that muscle will remain hiding behind a layer of body fat.

We already talked a lot about how muscle tone is essential for having an ideal Greek body. However, it is important to state that body fat plays a major role on how your body looks.

As mentioned in a previous chapter, the ancient Greeks were fanatics about having perfect body proportions.

Now keep this in mind…adding fat to any area of the body even a lit bit of fat will change your body ratios.

It is understandable that every person carries weight a little differently, leading to a couple of extra inches here and there.

For example, men that overeat tend to gain weight around their stomach and chest areas and women that overeat tend to gain weight around their hips and thighs.

In addition, we previously talked a little bit about the **3 body types** that people fit into which are **Ectomorph, Mesomorph and Endomorph**.

Ectomorphs are known as "hard gainers," because they can eat a lot of food but they have a hard time putting on weight.

Now, if you look at an **Endomorph**, it is very easy for them to gain weight so they have to be more cautious about what they eat.

It is important to state that your DIET is more important than exercise!

Many people believe that they can eat whatever they want and then easily burn those calories with exercise and this is simply not true.

Stop and think about how many calories are in some of your favorite foods.

Here are some examples of calories in different foods:

1. **A Big Mac has around 490 calories.** To burn those 490 calories, you will have to do 1 hour of intense strength training exercise or 42 minutes of intense cardio exercise.

2. **A pint of beer has 245 calories.** To burn off those 245 calories you would have to do 30 minutes of strength training exercise or 21 minutes of intense cardio exercise.

3. **2 slices of cheese pizza have around 600 calories.** To burn those 600 calories, you would have to swim 1 full hour to burn off those 2 slices of cheese pizza.

4. **4 small chocolate chip cookies have around 213 calories.** To burn those 213 calories, you would have to run 23 minutes on a treadmill.

5. **A small bag of potato chips has around 262 calories.** Now to burn those 262 calories you would have to walk 1 hour and 13 minutes.

6. **A small cup of vanilla and chocolate ice-cream has an estimated 540 calories.** Now to burn those 540 calories you would have to ride a bicycle for 1 hour and 22 minutes.

These examples of foods and their calorie amounts do not take into consideration all the other foods you eat on a daily basis as well as the amount of exercise you will need to do in order to burn those calories.

In order to truly obtain the physique of an ancient Greek warrior it is important to be mindful of your nutrition and eating habits. We will talk more about nutrition in the following chapters.

But for the moment, consider that although strength training exercises like bodyweight exercises will help you to build muscle it is also important to make cardio exercises part of your fitness training.

Making cardio exercises part of your fitness training is great for your body and health because cardio will help you to build stamina and reduce some of your bodyfat.

Although achieving a lean fit body is definitely a goal to aim at, it is important to state that having some body fat is actually good for your body and health.

For example, having small amounts of bodyfat is necessary for protecting your vital organs.

In addition, body fat provides your body with nutrients, gives you energy, helps with sport performance along with many other benefits.

Although you cannot completely eliminate bodyfat, you can definitely keep your bodyfat levels in check.

Keep this in mind…if you want to be lean, fit and functional, aim to have a low but healthy amount of bodyfat.

Having a low but healthy amount of bodyfat will give you a well-defined look to your physique.

So, want you want to do is tone and strengthen your entire body. In addition, you want to reduce some of your bodyfat with cardiovascular exercise.

As we have learned from ancient Greek art, the ideal Greek body was toned and lean, not weak and flabby.

It is important to state that the **ideal Greek bodyfat percentage** was about **10% fat** which is a good bodyfat percentage to have because it is low enough for displaying a toned, well-defined athletic body.

In addition, 10% bodyfat is quite a healthy bodyfat percentage to have because it is neither too low, nor too high.

Here is a chart showing bodyfat percentages for both men and women:

Ideal Bodyfat Percentage Chart

Description	Men	Women
Essential bodyfat	2-5% bodyfat (is not safe)	10-13% bodyfat (is not safe)
*Athletes	*6 - 13% bodyfat (is Ideal)	*14 - 20% bodyfat (is Ideal)

Casual Fitness	14-17% bodyfat	21-24% bodyfat
Average Person	18-24% bodyfat	24-31% bodyfat
Obese/Overweight	25% or more bodyfat	32% or more bodyfat

As you can see from the bodyfat percentage chart, having **6-13% bodyfat for men** and **14-20% bodyfat for women** is what you what to aim for when it comes to having an ideal bodyfat percentage.

Although the ideal bodyfat percentages for both men and women may seem difficult achieve it is important to state that it is greatly possible to achieve a low but healthy bodyfat percentage.

It addition, with hard work, good nutrition and making a commitment to get lean and fit, you can definitely achieve the goal of developing the body of an ancient Greek warrior.

As stated before, strength training will tone the body but cardiovascular exercise will "lean out" the body.

There are two types of cardiovascular exercises you want to include as part of your fitness training.

The first type is **aerobic exercise** and the second type is **anaerobic exercise**.

Aerobic exercise is any physical activity that consists of low intensity exercise that lasts for long periods of time.

For example, doing any physical exercise at a low intensity for 10, 20, 30 minutes or more would be considered aerobic exercise.

Some examples of aerobic exercise are running, swimming or cycling at a low intensity.

Now **anaerobic exercise** is intense, fast paced physical activity that is done in a short amount of time.

For example, running or swimming sprints at a full 100% capacity for very short distances are considered anaerobic exercises.

Anaerobic exercise is great for developing strength, speed and power whereas aerobic exercise is good for developing endurance.

Although some people may choose aerobic exercise over anaerobic exercise it is a good idea to do both in order to achieve the best weight loss results.

In addition, doing both aerobic and anaerobic exercise with make you more functional and athletic.

A great benefit of performing both aerobic and anaerobic exercises is that they will strengthen the heart and burn fat at the same time.

In order to get the best result for performing both aerobic and anaerobic exercises, it is a good idea to eat some healthy carbohydrates or "carbs."

Eating healthy carbohydrates will give your body the necessary energy it needs to perform both aerobic and anaerobic exercises effectively.

Although carbohydrates have developed a bad reputation in the past few years, many people seem too mix up the bad carbohydrates with the good carbohydrates.

Here is a short list of some good healthy carbohydrates that you want to eat:

<u>**Good Healthy Carbohydrates**</u>

1. Sweet Potatoes

2. Legumes, Lentils and Beans

3. Unprocessed Grains like Steel Cut Oats, Brown Rice and Quinoa

4. Fruits and Vegetables

Now that you know what carbohydrates are good for you to eat, lets look at a short list of some bad carbohydrates you want to stay away from:

<u>Bad Unhealthy Carbohydrates</u>

1. White bread

2. Bagels and Muffins

3. French Fries

4. Cakes and cookies

5. Sodas and Juices

As you can see from the list of bad unhealthy carbohydrates you want to stay away from, these are commonly eaten by many people.

What you want to do is try to only eat good healthy carbohydrates because they will give you the necessary energy and vitamins that your body needs for performing at your very best when it comes to cardiovascular exercise and overall exercise.

In addition, you want to remove unhealthy carbohydrates from your diet because they will make you gain weight and negatively affect your athletic performance.

As stated before, eating good healthy carbohydrates will give you the energy you need for performing at your very best when working out.

But something that is important to mention is that eating too many healthy carbohydrates can lead to weight gain especially if you don't use that energy.

So, what you want to do is make sure you only eat enough carbohydrates to fuel your workouts.

It is important to state that eating excess carbohydrates even excess protein can lead to weight gain so it is important to make sure you monitor your food intake.

One eating method that has become popular with many people that live a health and fitness lifestyle is the **Intermittent Fasting lifestyle**.

Living an Intermittent Fasting lifestyle while pursuing your goal of developing the physique of an ancient Greek warrior is a great idea.

You will be able to reduce your bodyfat percentage while developing a functional, athletic body as a result of practicing Intermittent Fasting.

In addition, you can even perform cardiovascular exercise while practicing Intermittent Fasting which will lead to rapid fat loss.

If you don't want to practice Intermittent Fasting but you want to make sure you are still able to burn fat effectively, then consider the Ketogenic Diet as an alternative.

The only downside to the Ketogenic Diet is that because it requires you to eat very few carbs, it is possible that you will not have enough energy for performing your strength training and cardiovascular exercises with 100% effort.

The one thing you can do is practice "Carb Cycling." "Carb Cycling" is simply alternating between low carb days and high carb days.

For example, if you are planning to run 7 miles today, then you would simply eat more carbohydrates today in order to have sufficient energy for your workout.

However, if you were planning to REST tomorrow and not do any exercise, you would then simply keep your carbohydrate intake low in order to prevent storing any excess calories from eating too many carbohydrates.

Keep in mind that both Intermittent Fasting and the Ketogenic Diet are great for controlling your weight and reducing fat loss.

In addition, combining strength training exercises with cardiovascular exercise will help you succeed at developing a body like an ancient Greek warrior.

You have already learned how strength training and cardiovascular exercise will help you to build strength and burn fat.

What I want to talk about now is a unique training method that can be used as a form of cardiovascular exercise.

This unique training method is called **Circuit Training**.

Circuit training is a method of training that requires you to perform one exercise after another with very little to no rest.

For example, look at the following Circuit Training Routine:

<u>**Bodyweight Circuit Routine**</u>

1. Bodyweight squats
2. Pushups
3. Bodyweight lunges
4. Pullups
5. Sit-ups
6. *rest 1 minute and repeat circuit 4 more times*

As you can see from this **Bodyweight Circuit Routine**, you are performing one bodyweight exercise immediately after another.

In addition, circuit training can be performed using machines, medicine balls, dumbbells and barbells.

Here are some other benefits of Circuit Training:

1. Works a lot of different muscles in the body.
2. Burns a lot of calories.
3. Provides a full body workout.
4. Allows you to exercise more in a short amount of time.
5. Develops strength and endurance.
6. Is fun and challenging.

What is great about **Circuit Training** is that you can perform between 4 through 8 **(4-8)** different exercises so that you can work different muscles of the body and get a total body workout.

In addition, you can perform between 6 through 12 **(6-12)** repetitions for each exercise when performing a **Circuit Training** routine.

This number of repetitions will help you to develop strength and improve your stamina as you aim to develop a lean, functional body like the ancient Greeks.

Here are a few more Circuit Training Routines you can use as a guide:

<u>Dumbbell Circuit Routine I</u>

1. Dumbbell deadlifts (6-12 Repetitions)
2. Dumbbell military press (6-12 Repetitions)
3. Dumbbells bent over rows (6-12 Repetitions)
4. Dumbbell squats (6-12 Repetitions)

rest 1 minute and repeat circuit 4 more times

<u>Bodyweight Circuit Routine II</u>

1. Pull-ups (6-12 Repetitions)
2. Jump Rope for 1 minute
3. Parallel Chest Dips (6-12 Repetitions)
4. Jump Rope for 1 minute

rest 1 minute and repeat circuit 4 more times

<u>Bodyweight Circuit Routine III</u>

1. Pull-up burpees (6-12 Repetitions)
2. Use Rowing machine for 1 minute
3. Dumbbell squat to shoulder press (6-12 Repetitions)
4. Use Rowing machine for 1 minute

rest 1 minute and repeat circuit 4 more times

***Alternate running in place or jump roping if there is no available rowing machine.*

It is important to state that starting a cardiovascular exercise routine, whether it is aerobic or anaerobic, is not difficult to do.

All you have to do is simply start off slow.

For example, if you want to start a running routine you can begin doing so by simply running at a slow to medium pace for 10 minutes, 4 days a week.

The following week you would then increase your running routine to 15 minutes, 4 days a week.

You can continue to slowly increase your running mileage until you feel comfortable enough to change up your running routine by doing some sprints.

By first running at a slow to moderate pace, which is consider **aerobic exercise**, you will be developing endurance.

After you have established a good running foundation, you can switch to running sprints, which is considered **anaerobic exercise**.

Remember, **anaerobic exercise** is great for developing strength, speed and power.

By performing both aerobic and anaerobic exercise, you will be developing endurance, strength and speed.

Overall, you will become more athletic and functional as a result of performing both aerobic and anaerobic exercise.

It is important to state that you want to start slow and increase your intensity slowly when beginning the process of doing aerobic and anaerobic exercises.

By starting slow and slowly increasing the intensity of your exercises, you will greatly reduce your chances of getting injured while exercising.

One final point to mention regarding cardiovascular exercise is **CONSISTENCY**.

Consistency is not only important with your cardiovascular exercises but also with your strength training exercises.

Consistency with your workouts is important because you want to continue to burn fat, get lean, improve with your workouts and remain motivated for achieving your health and fitness goals.

Keep this in mind, the minute you begin to skip a workout is the moment you develop the **HABIT** of making it ok to be inconsistent with your workouts.

In addition, being inconsistent with your workouts and simply foolishly skipping workouts can lead to a loss of motivation as well as a loss of strength and endurance which can lead to injury.

It is important to state that if you truly want to develop the physique like an ancient Greek warrior then you have to stay committed to living a health and fitness lifestyle.

Let me tell you, it is rewarding to achieve the body you want especially if you dedicate so much time, effort and discipline with your workouts and eating habits.

Developing a body like the ancient Greeks is something that not many people are willing to do because they are not willing to make a **Commitment** for doing so.

If you think about it, it is actually a lot easier to be **Average** and look like everyone else.

But ask yourself, "Do you want to be average?" "Do you want to look like everyone else?"

Some people may say that striving to develop a physique like the ancient Greeks is all about vanity but it is more, it is a lot more.

Through this process of developing your body, you will also be developing your **MIND**.

In addition, you will learn more about yourself then never before.

You will learn discipline, commitment, focus, sacrifice, determination, resilience, consistency, pain, suffering and achievement.

Now, it may take you 3, 6, 9 months or 1 year to achieve your lean, functional physique but you will achieve it if you are committed to achieving this goal and if you are consistent throughout the process.

In the end, when everything is said and done, you will have the body that you have been longing for.

Chapter 6: Your 8-Week Weight Training Guide

Before we begin, it is important to state that everybody will have a different starting point when it comes to beginning a weight training program.

As a result, it is important to tailor your weight training program according to your fitness levels.

The following weight training guide combines both strength training exercises as well as cardiovascular exercises.

Week one begins with half hour workouts that are meant to progress as weeks go on.

If you feel that starting with shorter workouts is better for your current fitness levels, then go ahead and cut the workouts in half.

The idea for the weight training program is for you to slowly progress and get stronger based on your current fitness levels.

In addition, you want to keep in mind that your weight training goal is to get stronger than you currently are and not to compete with others.

It is important to state that all the exercises that you will be performing for the weight training program will target all the muscle groups in the body.

In addition, be aware of any previous injuries you may have suffered and make sure to modify the weight training program as needed.

Remember you want to always think safety first when it comes to exercise.

As you look over the weight training program you will notice that there are only workouts scheduled for four or five days of the week.

The reason there are only workouts scheduled for four or five days of the week is because **Rest** and **Recovery** are very important in order for the body to repair itself and to avoid injury.

Actually, in the beginning you may even want to go ahead and modify the weight training program by resting more but it is important that you remain consistent with your training.

As stated before, tailor your weight training program according to your fitness levels.

Also, pay attention to how your body feels and if you feel your body needs more rest, then don't hesitate to take an extra day of rest.

Keep in mind that if you do rest more, this does not mean that you should simply sit down all day and do nothing.

Instead, you want to continue to exercise your heart and body by doing some easy exercise like walking.

Keep in mind that all weight training and weight bearing exercises are meant to be done slowly.

When performing an exercise, you want to make sure you take your time performing the exercise, have good form and really put in the necessary work for getting a great workout.

Week One: Determine your Baseline and Warm-up

This first week should be dedicated to finding out what your fitness levels are. You want to simply test your overall strength, agility and flexibility with various exercises.

Let's begin.

Week 1
You want to begin by doing a strength training workout on **day one**.

Then on **day two** you will do a cardiovascular workout.

Then on **day three** you will rest and recover.

So, you will follow this training schedule in the following order:
1. Day One – Strength Training
2. Day Two – Cardiovascular Workout
3. Day Three - Rest and Recover

Repeat this workout schedule routine, day after day, following the exact order throughout the entire 8-week training schedule.

Warm-up
You want to begin every strength training session with a 5-10-minute warm-up.
A warm-up can consist of the following body movements:

<u>**Warm-up Routine**</u>
1. Arm circles
2. Shoulder rotations
3. Neck circles
4. Waist rotations
5. Leg swings
6. 5-10 repetitions of Jumping jacks
7. Jog in place for 10-30 seconds

8. Feet shuffle side to side like a boxer for 10-30 seconds

repeat warm-up routine 2 to 3 times or as needed.

Here is your strength training workout routine for Week 1:

<u>**Strength Training Routine**</u>

1. Pushups
2. Bodyweight squats
3. Inverted rows or Chin-ups
4. Dumbbell Shoulder press (use light dumbbells)
5. Bodyweight Lunges

Rest for 1 minute and repeat the workout 4 more times
**Perform 6-12 repetitions for all exercises*

Here is your cardio workout for Week 1:

<u>**Cardio Routine**</u>

1. First, run or jog on a treadmill for 10 minutes
2. Next, ride a stationary bike for 10 minutes
3. Then, use a rowing machine for 10 minutes

Alternate between an elliptical machine or jump roping if an exercise machine is not available.

Here is how your workout schedule will look Monday through Sunday for Week 1:

Monday	Tuesday	Wednesday	Thursday	Friday	Saturday	Sunday
Strength Training Routine	Cardio Routine	***Rest and Recovery***	Strength Training Routine	Cardio Routine	***Rest and Recovery***	Strength Training Routine

As you can see from this training schedule, you will train two days consecutively which consists of one day of strength training followed by a second day of cardio exercise.

The third day is your rest and recovery day. On your rest day, you can do some "light" exercise like walking.

You will repeat this training cycle for the entire 8-week training program.

It is important to state that overworking your muscles can lead to decreased performance over time, extreme soreness and tiredness and can even lead to injury.

As a result, you can always modify the training schedule but remember to remain consistent with your workouts.

Weeks 2 and 3: Increase Intensity of Week One

Very simply, you will slowly increase the intensity of your workouts from week one by making the exercises more challenging.

In addition, there will be some new strength and cardio exercises included as part of your training for Weeks 2 and 3.

Remember to always warm-up before you begin your strength training routine.

Here is your strength training workout for Weeks 2 and 3:

<u>**Strength Training Routine**</u>

1. Decline Pushups   (Place both feet on a chair or bench and perform pushups)

2. Goblet squats (Use light weight)

3. Pull-ups   (Alternate between Pull-ups and Chin-ups)

4. Dumbbell shoulder press   (use light to moderate weight)

5. Dumbbell Lunges (use light weight)

Rest for 1 minute and repeat the workout 4 more times

Perform 6-12 repetitions for all exercises

Here is your cardio workout for Weeks 2 and 3:

<u>**Cardio Routine**</u>

1. First, jump rope for 10-15 minutes

2. Then, use a rowing machine for 10-15 minutes

3. Next, use an elliptical machine for 10-15 minutes

Alternate between a treadmill or stationary bike if an exercise machine is not available.

Here is how your workout schedule will look Monday through Sunday for Weeks 2 and 3:

Monday	Tuesday	Wednesday	Thursday	Friday	Saturday	Sunday
Strength Training Routine	Cardio Routine	*Rest and Recovery*	Strength Training Routine	Cardio Routine	*Rest and Recovery*	Strength Training Routine

Continue to follow your workout schedule of strength training day one, followed by doing cardio on day two, followed by resting on day three then repeating the cycle all over again on day four.

Continue to follow this workout schedule to make sure you build sustainable strength, stamina and for allowing your body to get enough rest.

Remember to do some "light" exercise on your "rest days" like walking.

Weeks 4 and 5: New Exercises and More Intensity

You will continue to increase the intensity of your workouts from the previous weeks by performing new exercises as well as increasing the intensity of your workouts.

In addition, you will perform "superset" routines for your strength training workouts.

"Supersets" are exercises that work opposing muscle groups. For example, chest and back exercises performed one right after the other are considered a "superset."

In addition, "Supersets" can also be exercises that work the upper and lower body by performing one exercise immediately after the other.

For example, performing a set of pushups for the upper body then immediately performing a set of bodyweight squats for the lower body will be considered a "superset."

Because you will be performing new exercises, you will be using some extra equipment in order to further challenge yourself as you progress with your workouts.

Here is your strength training workout for Weeks 4 and 5:

<u>**Strength Training Superset Routine I**</u>

    1. Weighted Chin-ups   (Use Light Weight)

    2. Explosive Jumping squats (Use 100% effort)

Rest for 1 minute and repeat the workout 4 more times

**Perform 6-12 repetitions for all exercises*

<u>**Strength Training Superset Routine II**</u>

    1. Parallel Dips Exercise

    2. Reverse Dumbbell Lunges (use light to moderate weight)

Rest for 1 minute and repeat the workout 4 more times

**Perform 6-12 repetitions for all exercises*

<u>**Strength Training Superset Routine III**</u>

    1. Dumbbell Shoulder Push Press   (use light to moderate weight)

    2. Mountain Climbers (use bodyweight)

Rest for 1 minute and repeat the workout 4 more times

**Perform 6-12 repetitions for all exercises*

Here is your cardio workout for Weeks 4 and 5:

<u>**Cardio Routine I**</u>

1. Perform Stair Running (Run up and down a flight of stairs for 30 seconds)

Rest for 1 minute and repeat the workout 10 more times

* Alternate Running every step, then running every other step.*

Cardio Routine II

1. First use a rowing machine for 10-15 minutes
2. Next, use an elliptical machine for 10-15 minutes

Alternate between a treadmill or stationary bike if an exercise machine is not available.

Weeks 6 and 7: Developing Strength, Endurance and Athleticism

By now, you should have developed some strength, speed, balance, agility, coordination, conditioning and flexibility.

Now you will continue to develop your strength, endurance and overall athleticism with more new and intense exercises.

Here is your strength training workout for Weeks 6 and 7:

Strength Training Routine I

1. Dumbbell Renegade Rows to Mountain Climbers (Use Light Weight)

Rest for 1 minute and repeat the workout 4 more times

**Perform 6-12 repetitions*

Strength Training Routine II

   1. Dumbbell squat to shoulder press   (Use Light Weight)

Rest for 1 minute and repeat the workout 4 more times

**Perform 6-12 repetitions*

Strength Training Routine III

   1. Pushups to Pull-ups Burpee

Rest for 1 minute and repeat the workout 4 more times

**Perform 6-12 repetitions*

Here is your cardio workout for Weeks 6 and 7:

Cardio Routine I

   1. Perform Stair Running Carrying light dumbbells or weights for 30 seconds

Rest for 1 minute and repeat the workout 10 more times

***Alternate Running every step, then running every other step.*

Cardio Routine II

   1. Perform 30 to 60-second Rowing Sprints

Rest for 1 minute and repeat the workout 10 more times

Alternate between a treadmill or stationary bike if an exercise machine is not available.

Cardio Routine III

   1. Use an elliptical machine for 10-15 minutes

Alternate between a treadmill or stationary bike if an exercise machine is not available.

Week 8: Test Yourself

You have come so far with your training. Now it is time to TEST your physical abilities.

It is important to state that the following tests only test a few specific exercises.

So, what you can do is test yourself using additional exercises if you like but simply use the following tests as a guide.

Keep in mind that before you test yourself, you want to make sure you properly warm-up.

In addition, you want to give yourself a few minutes to rest in between tests.

Here are the following tests you can use to measure your physical abilities:

Test #1 Pull-ups
You want to test yourself to see how many **pull-ups** you can do without stopping. Make sure to go all out and do your best!

Test #2 Parallel Dips Exercise
You want to test yourself to see how many **parallel dips** you can do without stopping. Make sure to go all out and do your best!

Test #3 Run 3 Miles for Time
You want to test yourself to see how **fast** you can **run 3 miles**. Use a stop watch to time yourself. In addition, make every effort to run as **fast** as possible.

After you complete the three tests determine if you need to improve your fitness levels.

If you realize that you do need to improve your fitness levels than simply retest yourself in 3 or 4 weeks.

One thing to keep in mind is that you always want to be improving with your workouts.

In addition, don't always do the same exercises and workouts months after months.

Instead, always be "evolving" with your workouts by trying new exercises and challenging yourself with new training equipment as well.

One final point I want to mention before we move on to the next chapter is the importance of stretching.

Stretching after you finish exercising whether it is completing a strength training session or a cardio workout is extremely important for the human body.

The kind of stretching you want to do after completing a tough workout is called "static stretching."

"Static stretching" is stretching a part of your body and holding this stretch for 30 seconds or more.

For example, holding onto a pull-up bar and hanging for 30 seconds would be considered "static stretching."

Another example of "static stretching" would be sitting down on the floor and reaching forward to touch your toes and holding this position for 30 seconds or more.

Here are some benefits of static stretching:

1. Improves your flexibility and the body's range of motion.

2. Reduces muscle soreness.

3. Corrects muscle imbalances of the joints.

4. Reduces risk of injury.

5. Improves athletic performance.

As you can see, stretching after completing a workout is very important for the body.

Try to do between 10 and 15 minutes of stretching after working out in order to "cool down" and relax the body and mind.

Chapter 7: Ancient Greek Nutrition

Working out hard is important and easy to do.

But what is very difficult for many people to do is to properly fuel their bodies with the right foods.

In order to perform at your best when working out, you have to eat the right foods in order to properly fuel your body.

In addition, in order to burn fat, get lean and build muscle you have to discipline yourself to follow a healthy eating plan.

Because you want to build a lean functional physique like the ancient Greeks, let's look at nutrition through the eyes of the ancient Greeks themselves.

For example, the ancient Greeks ate bread dipped in wine for breakfast whereas modern day breakfast consists of drinking sugary juice and eating bacon and maybe some eggs or a bagel.

For lunch the ancient Greeks would eat more bread dipped in wine but it also included eating dried fish, olives, figs and cheese.

For the ancient Greeks, dinner was the main meal of the day consisting of fish, vegetables and fruit.

To give their food some flavor, the ancient Greeks would use natural honey as a way to sweeten their food.

The ancient Greeks were known to eat a lot of fish. In addition, fish was the main source of protein for the ancient Greeks.

However, the amount of fish and meat an ancient Greek person would eat would depend on how wealthy they were.

Beef was rarely eaten because it was very expensive and pork was eaten by poor Greeks and slaves.

It is important to state that the ancient Greeks ate very little meat especially when you compare how much meat is consumed every day in developed nations.

The ancient Greeks were considered "frugal" with their food. Only the wealthy would indulge in eating lots of meat and beef.

The ancient Greeks were known for consuming a lot of wine. However, the wine would be "watered down" and was consumed slowly.

Milk was not consumed by the ancient Greeks but instead it was used for producing cheese.

Because the ancient Greeks did not have forks, spoons or knives to use for eating, they would simply eat with their hands.

In addition, the ancient Greeks would use bread to eat their soup by scooping it up using the bread.

It can be said that the ancient Greeks ate a lot of bread and the two main grains they used for making bread were wheat and barley.

For the ancient Greeks, fruits and vegetables were a very important part of their diet.

The ancient Greeks would include a lot of vegetables in their soups. In addition, foods like lentil soup were very popular with the ancient Greeks.

An everyday working Greek man would eat a lot of lentil soup and garlic and a Greek soldier's main source of food consisted of onions and cheese.

Fruits and nuts were eaten as desserts. The most important fruits for the ancient Greeks were pomegranates, raisons and dried figs.

Ancient Greek warriors like the Spartans would mostly eat a "black soup" or "black broth" made up of boiled pork, pig's blood, vinegar and salt.

This "black soup" the Spartans would eat was a staple food for them because they believed it would give them extreme strength and power.

In addition, this "black soup" the Spartans would eat was served with dried figs and cheese and if they were lucky, sometimes they would get to eat some fish or other animal.

Now those Greeks that lived along the coastline would eat a lot of fresh fish and seafood.

In addition, foods like sardines and anchovies were very popular with those Greeks that lived along the coastline.

Another important food the ancient Greeks would eat were eggs.

Greeks ate eggs specifically from hens and quails. In addition, eggs were often eaten as appetizers or dessert.

Another important food that was a staple food for the ancient Greeks was cheese.

Cheese was often eaten with honey and vegetables.

In addition, nuts like walnuts and almonds were very popular with the ancient Greeks.

And when it comes to water, the ancient Greeks would drink a lot of "spring water" which was always preferred over water from wells.

After water, wine was their drink of choice. The ancient Greeks would sometimes sweeten their wine with honey.

There were also religious Greeks that practiced vegetarianism with some Greeks restricting themselves to only eating bread and water.

Ancient Greeks would also use a lot of herbs in their cooking and meals.

The ancient Greeks did not complicate their meals but instead simply ate what was available to them.

Now that you know a little about what the ancient Greek people used to eat, lets focus now on what the ancient Greek Athletes used to eat.

Greek Athletes

Ancient Greek athletes ate simple foods. If they could afford it, they would eat meat but fish was the preferred source of protein for Greek athletes.

In addition, Greek athletes ate a lot of dried fruit. For example, dried figs were a main source of food for the ancient Greek athletes.

Greek athletes would practice the importance of having a healthy diet especially if they were to participate in the Olympic Games.

Usually, an athlete's diet would consist of foods such as fresh cheese, bread and dried figs.

Some athletes were even instructed to eat more meat and follow a "meat diet" which consisted of eating a lot of meat for the purpose of getting stronger.

For example, there was this very famous Olympic champion wrester that was considered to be the greatest wrestler of ancient Greece.

He was known to eat 20 pounds of meat per day! In addition, he would eat several pounds of bread every day as well as drink lots and lots of wine on a daily basis.

Now this ancient Greek wrestler was the exception and not the norm.

But overall, Greek athletes were known for eating a healthy balanced diet and they were very careful about the foods they ate.

Greek athletes also had trainers that would teach them about the importance of having a healthy diet.

For example, athletic trainers would instruct the Greek athletes to stay away from desserts and from drinking wine.

Greek athletes would also eat bread, specifically flatbread which was made of barley or wheat.

Although the amount of wine a Greek athlete would consume during training was reduced or eliminated, they still enjoyed consuming their wine.

In addition, Greek athletes loved olive oil.

It can be said that Greek athletes truly enjoyed consuming olive oil so much that some athletes went as far as bathing themselves in olive oil before a fitness competition.

It is important to mention that just as there are different food diets and food trends today, there were also food trends during ancient Greece times.

For example, if there was a Greek athlete that stated he did not eat bread for whatever reason, then other people would soon follow this "no bread" diet.

Another food trend that was popular with Greek athletes was the "raw honey" diet.

There were some Greek athletes that believed that consuming lots of raw honey would give them lots of energy for making them top performing athletes.

However, after some years, other Greek athletes would practice the "no honey" diet because they believed the sugar in honey would make them slow.

What is interesting about these food trends during ancient Greece was that Greek athletes were not looking for a food trend to follow but instead they were seeking to improve their diets with a sense of "perfection" and "purity."

It can be said that the diet of ancient Greek athletes was simple consisting of fish, bread, olive oil and wine.

However, the Greek athletes placed great importance on eating the best and purest sources of food that would help them to succeed in their sport and in the Olympic Games.

As you can recall from the previous chapters, the ancient Greeks believed a lot in "perfection."

The Greek athletes wanted to eat the perfect foods and have the perfect diet and the Greeks in general believed in having ideal perfect physiques.

Even the Greek statues were created with great perfection by its sculptors.

Even the Greek farmers strived to grow perfect crops for the athletes and for the general Greek population to eat.

The ancient Greeks were definitely perfectionists.

Food and The Olympic Games

Before we continue to learn more about Greek athletes and their eating habits let's look at a brief history regarding the Olympic Games:

1. Ancient Olympia is the birthplace of the Olympic Games.
2. The first Olympic Games were held in 776 B.C.
3. The Olympic Games were meant to honor Zeus, the God of Sky and Thunder and King of the Gods.
4. Only men were allowed to attend and watch the Olympic Games.

It is important to state that Greek athletes that were participating in the Olympic games were required to travel long distances by foot or sea to the small city village of Olympia.

Because the village of Olympia was so small, it did not have enough food to feed all the athletes as well as all the people that would go to watch the Olympic Games.

So, many athletes, with the help of farmers, would package nothing but the best and healthiest foods and carry this food with them to the Olympic Games.

The Greek athletes were also required to bring enough food to last the long journey to the Olympic Games from their hometowns.

The Greek athletes also had to bring enough food to eat during the Olympic Games.

They Greek athletes also had to bring enough food to eat for the giant celebration that followed the conclusion of the Olympic Games.

And the Greek athletes still had to make sure they had enough food for their trip back to their hometowns after the Olympic Games were over.

As you can see, the ancient Greeks were not only athletes but also true warriors.

It can be said that Greek athletes developed a mental toughness mindset of surviving on little food yet competing at the highest levels in sports competition for honor and glory.

Because the Olympic Games and training as an athlete for the Olympic Games were very important, the farmers were always making sure to grow the best foods for the Greek athletes.

In addition, the farmers made every effort to prepare food for the Greek athletes well in advanced for the Olympic Games.

In addition, the farmers were very proud of the foods they grew for the Greek athletes.

The farmers believed that if a Greek athlete was victorious at the Olympic Games it was because they were growing the best foods.

What can be said of ancient Greek athletes is that they spent years perfecting their diets as well as transporting their food from their hometowns to the Olympic Games.

With the help of farmers, Greek athletes made sure to eat nothing but the best foods they could feed their bodies.

And if Greek athletes were to become victorious during the Olympic Games, it was because of the foods they ate.

Now that you know a little about what ancient Greek athletes ate to perform at their highest levels, let's look at how you too can eat like an ancient Greek athlete.

Eating Like the Ancient Greeks

It has been said that if you want to be successful at something, do what successful people do.

So, if you want to develop a lean, functional physique like the ancient Greeks then simply eat and train like the ancient Greeks.

Exercising and training especially in modern times is very easy to do because we have access to all kinds of gyms, fitness equipment, online exercise videos and fitness apps to help us with our workouts.

But the hard part of developing a lean, functional physique is not the exercise part but rather following a healthy diet every day for 3, 6, 9 months or 1 year.

If you can practice eating a healthy diet every day for several months than you will be successful at developing an athletic physique like the ancient Greeks.

What is important to remember is that developing a lean functional physique like the ancient Greeks is all about living a health and fitness lifestyle.

Therefore, you have to make living a health and fitness lifestyle a **priority** in your life if you truly want to develop a lean, functional physique.

You already learned that following a healthy diet for the ancient Greeks was very important.

Therefore, it is going to be just as important for you to also follow a healthy diet especially now more than ever because of the easy access we have to processed and unhealthy foods.

You want to always keep in mind to do as the ancient Greeks did and that is to keep your diet simple and focus on eating natural healthy foods.

Consider the following foods for eating simple, natural, healthy foods:

1. For eating healthy sources of protein, focus on eating fish and chicken.

2. For eating vegetables, consider eating spinach, lettuce and broccoli.

3. For eating healthy carbohydrates, consider eating legumes and sweet potatoes.

4. For eating healthy fats, consider eating avocados and healthy nuts like almonds and walnuts.

5. To add flavor to your food, consider using lemon, spicy hot sauce or some low calorie sweet sauce.

As you can see from this simple but natural food list, eating healthy does not have to be difficult.

You just have to make a commitment to eating healthy followed by creating a plan regarding the types of foods you plan to eat.

Chapter 8: Health Benefits of Eating and Training Like the Ancient Greeks

The goal of eating and training like the ancient Greeks is not just to have a great body, but to live a healthier life.

In addition, by eating natural healthy foods and making exercise part of your daily life, you will be 10 times healthier than the majority of people.

It is important to state that by developing a naturally lean and powerful body like the ancient Greeks, you will develop confidence and discipline within yourself.

In addition, you will come to know what pain and sacrifice are.

You will develop mental toughness and a winning mindset to succeed at achieving your goals.

You will develop tremendous patience and focus especially in a time when everyone wants to lose 10 pounds in 1 day.

Let me tell you this journey of developing a lean, functional physique is not going to be easy nor fast but the process and the end goal are well worth it.

It can be stated that after several months of staying committed to eating healthy and training hard, you will feel victorious just like the ancient Greek athletes felt victorious when they succeeding at winning at the Olympic Games.

It is important to state that going through the process of developing a lean, functional physique is an excellent goal to achieve but what is more important is what you will become as a result of achieving this goal.

You will become a "role model" to others of how to live, eat and train like a modern-day warrior.

People will look up to you and ask you about how they too can achieve their health and fitness goals.

Remember, you are not seeking to be a bodybuilder but instead you are seeking to develop a lean, functional physique.

It is important to state that many people are looking for "shortcuts" to achieving their health and fitness goals by taking all kinds of supplements, steroids and other stimulants.

However, it is very important that you stay away from all of these supplements and stimulants and remain "natural" because all of those supplements and stimulants will negatively affect your overall health later in life.

Keep in mind that the idea of creating an ideal Greek body is all about achieving good health the natural way.

In order to benefit from eating healthy and training like the ancient Greeks, you must truly embrace this lifestyle

Keep in mind that the ancient Greeks lived in a very different time than we currently live in today.

The ancient Greeks lived in an era before there were so many modern conveniences like easy access to all kinds of foods, supermarkets and fast food restaurants that deliver food in 30-minutes or less.

In addition, the ancient Greeks were a lot busier than people are today.

For example, there was no time for a Greek person to sit around and surf the internet, watch television or play video games because computers and televisions had not yet been invented.

Instead, the ancient Greeks were active in their communities as well as busy working as farmers or they would simply be out enjoying nature.

There were also those ancient Greeks that stayed busy by training religiously to be soldiers, warriors and Olympic athletes.

Should you decide to embrace the ancient Greek lifestyle and live with the purpose of creating a body that is both healthy and functional, your health and overall quality of life will greatly improve.

If you need more reasons to embrace the ancient Greek warrior lifestyle then consider the following 11 benefits of living this amazing lifestyle:

1. Regular exercise and eating healthy both improve your mood and give you tremendous energy.

2. Exercise and eating healthy fight off diseases and illnesses and prevent obesity.

3. Exercise and healthy eating improve your quality of sleep and extend your lifespan.

4. Exercise and healthy eating improve your levels of productivity at work and in your overall life.

5. Exercise and healthy eating help you to look and feel younger.

6. Eating healthy and physical exercise help you to focus better, improve your memory, make you more alert and improve your brain power making you smarter.

7. Eating healthy and doing exercise will strengthen you heart, body and mind.

8. Exercise and eating healthy will reduce stress and help you to relax more.

9. Eating healthy and physical exercise will improve your confidence and help you to be more creative.

10. Exercise and eating healthy can be fun, social and improve your sex life.

11. Physical exercise and eating healthy can help you to develop discipline, commitment, focus, patience and determination.

As you can see, there are so many benefits of why living a healthy and fitness lifestyle like the ancient Greeks is so rewarding.

Sure, it will be difficult at times especially in the beginning and sure, it will take time to burn some fat and get fit but so what.

Simply, EVERYTHING TAKES TIME!

Make a positive step in your life by committing to living a health and fitness lifestyle for the next eight weeks.

After eight weeks, evaluate your results by asking yourself the following questions:

1. "How much fat did I burn?"

2. "How much stronger did I get?"

3. "How do I feel after eight weeks of living a health and fitness lifestyle?"

4. "How has my quality of life improved?"

Even after eight weeks of training and eating healthy, consider making living a health and fitness lifestyle a permanent goal.

Keep in mind that your health and fitness lifestyle does not have to be perfect but you do have to be consistent with your workouts and with maintaining your healthy eating habits.

Remember, you are human so you will make mistakes along your health and fitness journey.

However, never be discouraged and always remember that you are living a positive and rewarding health and fitness lifestyle the ancient Greek way.

Conclusion

Thanks for making it through to the end of *Bodybuilding: How to Build the Body of a Greek God.*

This book has been about more than just creating the body of a Greek God.

This book has taught you about how the ancient Greeks lived, ate and trained on a daily basis.

This book has also taught you how the ancient Greeks saw the human body as a beautiful art form.

Now that you have come to learn the overall lifestyle that ancient Greek warriors lived in order to achieve their ideal physiques, it is now time for you to go out and live that same lifestyle.

Remember, the ancient Greeks were active members of society. They used brute strength and stamina on a daily basis and developed their lean, athletic bodies without even trying.

In addition, the ancient Greeks followed a very healthy but simple diet that consisted of natural foods they grew and raised themselves.

So, if you are looking to develop a body like a Greek God, then you must learn to adjust your lifestyle to one that supports and maintains your physique.

Hopefully, this book was informative and was able to provide you with all of the tools you need to achieve your goal of developing a lean, functional physique.

Remember, developing a lean, functional physique is a process and it will take hard work and commitment.

Therefore, use the information you have learned in this book and make a commitment to transform your body and your life.

Tips for Rapid Fat Loss

Below are 30 of the Best Tips for Rapid Fat Loss.

Tip #1 Learn to Cook Healthy Food in Under 20 minutes

Believe it or not but you can learn to cook healthy food in under 20 minutes!

In order to cook healthy food in under 20 minutes it is important to follow the **Kiss Principal** which stands for:

K=Keep
I=It
S=Simple
S=Stupid

Here are four great, easy to make recipes that you can use for cooking healthy food in under 20 minutes:

Recipe 1 (Chicken Fajitas)

- Chop chicken breast into small pieces and cook high on a pan for 10-15 minutes.

- Serve chopped chicken with precooked sweet potatoes that are reheated.

- Include a large bowl of washed lettuce with your meal.

*Add some low sodium hot sauce to your Chicken Fajitas for some spicy flavor.

Recipe 2 (Breakfast/Lunch Oats)

- Use Sugar Free Oatmeal or Steel Cut Oats.
- Boil Hot Water for 5-10 Minutes.
- Pour hot water onto bowl of oatmeal and stir for 2 or 3 minutes.
- Serve Oatmeal with Frozen Greek Yogurt.
  *Add blueberries, almonds or cashews to your Oatmeal

Recipes 3 (Scrambled Eggs with Avocado)

1. Cook 3 or 4 whole scrambled eggs.
2. Serve eggs with 1 large avocado (feel free to mix avocado with eggs).
3. Include a large bowl of washed spinach with your meal.
   *Desert can be some blackberries, walnuts and dark chocolate

Recipe 4 (Fish and Veggies)

- Open 1 or 2 cans of tuna.
- Serve with low sodium whole wheat crackers.
- Include frozen mixed veggies or spinach.
  *Add some low sodium sauce to your tuna.

Tip #2 Cook For 2 or 3 Days!

When you cook, consider cooking enough healthy food to last you 2 or 3 days.

Cooking enough food to last you 2 or 3 days will definitely save you a lot of time!

Consider cooking simple foods like chicken breasts, which can be cooked in under 20 minutes and save the leftovers in the refrigerator.

You can also boil multiple sweet potatoes while at home and save any leftovers in the fridge.

What is great about boiling sweet potatoes is that they are extremely healthy for you and they involve No Cooking whatsoever!

Cooking enough healthy food to last you 2 or 3 days is a great way to make sure you always have something healthy to eat no matter how busy you are.

In addition, cooking enough food that last you 2 or 3 days is a great way to cut down on the amount of time you spend cooking and cleaning in the kitchen.

Tip # 3 Order Your Groceries from The Internet

If you hate going to a crowded supermarket or your simply just too busy to go grocery shopping then consider shopping for groceries online!

Here are some advantages of shopping for groceries online:

Convenience: You don't have to wait in long lines to purchase your groceries. Instead, you can do your grocery shopping online in minutes. Plus, you can shop for your groceries 24 hours a day, 7 days a week!

Better Prices: You can sometimes get better prices from online grocery stores because they want more and more people to use their services.

In addition, some online grocery stores may even offer coupons and free home delivery.

Fewer Expenses: You don't have to pay for gas for your car when you shop for groceries online.

You don't even need to own a car to shop online! Instead you can simply save money by not having a car and by simply shopping for your groceries online and having them delivered directly to your home.

Delivery to Your Front Door: You don't have to worry about going out in the snow, rain or during busy rush hour traffic to purchase groceries.

You can instead simply order your groceries online and simply have them delivered to your home for a small free and sometimes for free!

No Unwanted Unhealthy Food: It's far too easy to walk into a supermarket and be tempted to buy unhealthy food.

Instead, buying groceries online simply allows you to buy exactly what you need without having any temptations to purchase additional foods especially all those delicious looking deserts that are usually placed at the entrance of supermarkets.

Tip #4 Use The 80/20 Rule

The 80/20 Rule is a very simple principle that goes like this: 80% of the time eat healthy and 20% of the time eat whatever you want and this could include your favorite dessert.

For example, let's say you eat a healthy dinner that consists of skinless chicken breasts, boiled sweet potatoes and a bowl of spinach.

If you decide to include a small bowl of chocolate ice-cream then you now just made dessert part of your dinner.

So, around 80% of your dinner consisted of healthy foods such as chicken breasts, sweet potatoes and spinach and the other 20% consisted of your chocolate ice-cream dessert which is not considered a top healthy food choice.

If you apply the 80/20 Rule to your eating habits, you will develop the habit of eating healthy 80% percent of the time while you give yourself some space to enjoy some of your favorite desserts and foods 20% of the time.

Tip # 5 Eliminate or Limit Your Alcohol Intake

Plain and simple…alcohol, especially beer makes you fat!

The more beer you drink that fatter you will get. In addition, drinking alcohol especially beer can make you hungry causing you too eat unhealthy fast food.

As a result, limit your alcohol intake or completely eliminate it.

If you are going to drink, consider drinking a small glass of red wine.

Tip #6 Avoid Overeating With "Portion Control"

Overeating can cause weight gain, even if you are eating healthy foods.

However, you can prevent excess weight gain from overeating by practicing "portion control."

"Portion control" is simply reducing the amount of food you eat by eating smaller portions.

The best way to reduce the amount of food you eat is by using a small food scale. You can also consider using a smaller bowl or plate for reducing the amount of food you eat.

However, using a food scale for reducing the amount of food you eat is 100% more accurate than using a small bowl or plate.

When it comes to "portion control" using a food scale, all you have to do is simply weigh your food before you eat it so that you will know exactly how much food you are consuming for each meal.

So, if you want to simply lose a few extra pounds all you have to do is simply reduce the amount of food you are eating by using your food scale.

The concept of "portion control" is very popular with bodybuilders, weightlifters and competitive athletes.

Nutritionists are also known to recommend their clients to use "portion control" as a way of reducing obesity.

Tip #7 Eat Natural Foods

To lose weight, stay healthy and keep your energy levels high as you strive to be a successful in life, it is very important to eat natural foods.

Why eat natural foods?

Because, foods like fruits, vegetables, nuts, lean cuts of meat and healthy fats have a lot of vitamins and minerals that are excellent for providing the body and mind with optimal health.

Here are some more benefits of eating Natural Foods:

- Natural foods will help boost your energy levels for optimal performance giving you superior energy to work harder and smarter.

- Natural foods are great for fighting off chronic diseases and illness as well as for preventing you from getting sick.

- Natural foods like fruits and veggies are low calorie water foods that will supply your body with a lot of water and fiber and will help you to feel full and eat less.

- Because natural foods are healthier for you, they will help you to lose weight.

Keep in mind that the more natural foods you eat, the more weight you will lose.

In addition, you will have more energy, feel healthier and be able to perform at your best as a result of eating more natural foods.

Tip #8 Practice Intermittent Fasting

Intermittent fasting is a very effective healthy eating method that any busy person can incorporate into their busy lives.

Intermittent fasting works by eating within a certain time period or an "eating window" within a day and then fasting for the rest of the day.

For example, let's say you have an "eating window" Monday - Friday from 11:00 AM – 7:00 PM.

This means that you can eat (usually 1 or 2 meals or more) from 11:00 AM – 7:00 PM. Once your "eating window" closes, you simply fast for the rest of the day.

When you temporarily fast for a period of time, you get to experience all kinds of benefits.

Some of The Benefits of Intermittent Fasting Are:

- You develop discipline with your eating habits.
- You will feel very alert and energetic while fasting.
- Increases your life expectancy.
- Helps you to lose weight and hunger.
- Allows you to develop a flexible eating schedule around your busy work/life.

- Allows you to eat only 1 or 2 meals a day giving you more free time to focus on other priorities.

Overall, intermittent fasting is a great tool that any busy person can use for eating healthy and staying fit.

Tip #9: Use A Food Journal

Using a food journal is a great way to keep track of all the food you eat on a daily basis.

All you have to do is simply write down what eat you every day. Make sure to include any snacks, teas, coffee and drinks in your food journal.

Writing down what you eat using a food journal is a great habit to develop. You will come to realize how healthy you are eating as well as all the unhealthy foods you may be eating.

In addition, you can look back at all the food you ate on any given day and determine whether you ate too much.

If you feel like you are simply eating too much or that you want to lose a few pounds, you can use your food journal as a way to see what foods you may want to eat less of.

You can keep track of the food you eat by using notebook, or you can use your computer or you can even use an app.

Using a food journal is great for helping you to keep focused on your diet, helps you to develop good eating habits, provides motivation for achieving your health and fitness goals and it is an efficient way to simply burn fat and lose weight.

At the end of the day, you can refer back to your food journal and ask yourself questions like:

Did I eat a healthy delicious meal?

Did I eat enough fruits and vegetables?

Did I drink enough water?

Did I eat any unhealthy foods or snacks?

Didi I feel extremely full after each meal?

Did I feel energetic or tired as a result of the foods I ate?

Tip #10 Drink Lots of Water Every Day!

Water is great for the body. But did you know that foods such as a fruits and vegetables are not only full of vitamins and minerals, but they are also full of water?

Simply drinking more water and eating more water foods on a daily basis has so many benefits such as:

- Water gives you lots of energy.

- Water is great for your skin.

- Water prevents you from feeling fatigue as a result of dehydration.

- Water helps you to feel full.

- Prevents you from feeling hungry.

- Helps reduce weight loss.

- Is great for your ligaments, tendons and joints. So, water lubricates your body!

Eating more fruits and vegetables on a daily basis is high recommended not only for the vitamins and nutrients they provide but also for the amount of water they provide.

As a result, don't underestimate the power of water!

Water is magical!

Tip #11 Remove All Junk Food from Your Home

Simply, remove all junk food from your home and instead replace these unhealthy foods with healthy snacks.

Some healthy snacks to eat are fruits and healthy nuts like almonds, walnuts and cashews and you can even eat some dark chocolate!

If you are a busy working professional, consider taking healthy snacks to your office instead of buying unhealthy foods and snacks on the way to work.

Tip #12 Take A Break Every Hour

Simply take a break every hour from sitting down and get your body moving.

You can take a break for 10-15 minutes and maybe do some light stretching or you can even do some dynamic stretches like arm and leg circles as well as hip and waist rotations.

You can even do some easy body-weight exercises like push-ups, body-weight squats or lunges to get the blood flowing in your body.

Tip #13 Set A Schedule and Develop Discipline to Stick to It

Some people are morning people and others are night owls. Do whatever works best for you.

However, develop the habit of creating a work, eating and fitness schedule and stick to it so that you can make sure you are living a healthy lifestyle.

In addition, developing a work, eating and fitness schedule will keep you focused on what is important and what you should focus on as well as what your priorities are.

You will also be more organized if you develop a work, eating and fitness schedule and stick to it than if you had no plan whatsoever.

Tip #14 Create a Healthy Environment

Whether you work from home or from your work office, create an environment that is relaxing and enjoyable for you.

You can look into getting some home/office fitness gear such as a work desk to make sure you are moving your body or you can even use a gym chair which provides a total body workout.

You can even consider getting a cycling work station or a under desk treadmill for the purpose of getting some exercise while you work or watch TV at home.

Tip #15 Sleep More

According to research, sleep is more important than nutrition and exercise.

A lack of sleep will reduce your mental and physical performance. In addition, lack of sleep will develop stress in your body causing you to gain weight.

A lack of sleep will also affect your mood and hormones.

As you can see, you want to make sure you sleep as much as possible especially if you want to burn fat effectively.

Sleep is extremely beneficial for being successful in overall life because it will repair your body and mind from all the mental and physical stress you put it through day after day so make sure you are getting lots and lots of sleep.

I will talk more about the importance of sleep and its benefits later.

Tip #16 Plan Your Meals and Eat the Same Meals

Plan your meals ahead. You can also develop the habit of eating the same healthy foods every day both for lunch and dinner.

This keeps shopping for healthy foods easy and it is an efficient way of eating because you will develop the habit of shopping for and cooking the same foods every day.

Tip # 17 Use A Food Scale

Use a food scale to weigh your food before you cook it so that you know exactly how much food you will be consuming every day both for lunch and dinner.

By using a food scale, you will be able to keep track of the number of calories you are eating every day.

In addition, you will be more efficient at losing weight because you will not be overeating as a result of keeping track of how much food you eat.

Research shows that 80% of weight loss is all about your diet and what you eat and how much you eat.

So, by weighing your food, you will know if you need to reduce the number of calories you are eating in order to lose weight.

In addition, weighing your food will help you to maintain your desired weight.

Tip #18 Develop a Health and Fitness Calendar

The same way you have appointments, meetings and deadlines for your work and personal life is the same way you should have them also for your health and fitness goals.

Simply develop a schedule on your calendar that allows you to have time for exercise, rest and recreation.

Developing a health and fitness calendar will help you to break away from your daily routine.

Making health and fitness a priority is a great way to make sure you are giving your body and mind a break from all the stress and challenges you face on a daily basis.

In addition, you will feel more energetic, focused and productive as a result of taking the time to exercise and improve your well-being.

You will also have positive energy, a lot of focus and high levels of productivity that will help you to continue to succeed in losing weight and achieving your personal goals.

So, use a calendar and schedule your workouts, schedule your breaks, schedule your yoga classes, schedule your meals, simply prioritize scheduling your health and fitness lifestyle.

Tip #19 Exercise More

Try to squeeze more exercise into your daily life.

Begin your day with an early walking routine.

Consider working out at home if you are really too busy to make it to the gym.

Whatever you do, try to move more throughout the day because you will feel less fatigue then if you just sit down at a desk all day.

Research shows that exercise improves your ability to think better. In addition, exercise will make you happier and feel better.

Here are some other ways that exercise will improve not only your health but also your mind:

- Increases your level of focus.

- Improves your memory.

- Develops discipline and focus.

- Improves your work performance and time management skills.

- Improves your immune system which means you will not get sick as often.

- Gives you more energy to do more especially when it comes to achieving your health and fitness goals and any other personal goals.

As you can see exercise strongly affects how well you will succeed in your overall life.

As a result, develop an exercise plan and stick to it so that you can experience great results in both your health and in overall life.

Tip #20 Eat More Vegetables, Fish and Fruits

Eat healthier to look and feel better. When you look and feel better you will feel more confident in yourself to achieve more in life.

Simply eating lots of fresh vegetables and fruits will give you all the energy you need to succeed in life and with achieving your health and fitness goals.

In addition, you have to include fish in your diet because it is good for the heart, good for the joints, improves your mood, strengthens your immune system, it improves your sleep and more!

It is important to state that people that eat healthy have higher levels of productivity.

In addition, a person's physical work capacity and performance is greatly increased as a result of eating a healthier diet.

If you still don't think that eating healthy is important than consider this: **research shows that the amount of money that you make is a result of your eating habits.**

So, the healthier you eat the more money you are likely to make. However, if you have a poor diet, then you will simply be poor.

Tip #21 Write Down Everything

Write down your financial goals, your fitness goals, your life goals, write down all your goals and try to slowly accomplish them little by little every day.

You will feel better when you see what you are accomplishing every day by writing down what you achieve every day.

In addition, you will have a better understanding of what areas you need to improve on.

You can refer back to your daily accomplishments knowing that you did everything you could to succeed and as a result you will sleep better.

The next day when you wake up, you will wake up energetic, hungry and ready to get started on your daily projects and goals to see how much you can accomplish.

You will eventually develop healthy habits like drinking more water, sleeping more and getting more exercise as you continue to write down your daily goals and reflect on your accomplishments.

You will come to learn how sleeping more, drinking more water and daily exercise are important for accomplishing any goal in life.

You will soon have a full daily schedule prioritizing your health, work and life goals eliminating everything that is unimportant in life.

As you continue to remain focus on your daily schedule, you will succeed at achieving your goals as a result of developing priorities for achieving your health and fitness and other goals.

You will develop a lot more focus in life as a result of writing down your goals.

So, track your weight loss progress and other goals you want to achieve and be aware if things are working or if you need to make some changes.

Tip # 22 Use A Fitness Tracker

If you are a busy person that wants to exercise, eat healthy and feel great but needs some motivation to get stared and remain motivated, then consider using a fitness tracker.

What is a Fitness Tracker?

A fitness tracker is a cool looking device that is more like a small computer that you wear around your wrist like a watch.

Fitness trackers can monitor and track your health and fitness related activities like keeping count of your running mileage as well as how many calories you have burned.

Fitness trackers can even monitor your sleep as well as your heart rate and more!

Overall, fitness trackers are great for motivating you to get in shape as well as stay in shape.

Here are some more ways fitness trackers can help you achieve your health and fitness goals:
- Keep track of your daily health and fitness progress.

- Provide free workouts and tips.

- Help you set achievable fitness goals.

- Monitor your sleep patterns and breathing.

- Assist you with developing healthy habits like walking more and eating less.

- Send alerts to remind you to get up and move more.

- Monitors your diet, calories, and the foods you eat.

- Assists with training for a marathon and burning fat.

What is great about fitness trackers is that they act like a personal trainer that is always conveniently available to you 24 hours a day, 7 days a week, 365 days a year.

Overall, fitness trackers are one of the best ways to make sure you achieve your health and fitness goals.

Tip #23 Use A Fitness App

Research show that people that use fitness apps are likelier to remain consistent with their health and fitness lifestyle then people that don't use fitness apps.

In addition, research also shows that people that use fitness apps are more active than people that don't use fitness apps.

As you can see, fitness apps are great for keeping you in shape. In addition, there are all kinds of fitness apps that you can use from running apps to strength training apps to yoga apps to even nutrition apps.

Overall, fitness apps are great for making sure you stay consistent with your health and fitness lifestyle.

Tip #24 Make A Commitment to Exercise

It is important to be consistent with getting some exercise every day no matter how busy you may be.

Simply, don't make excuses for not be able to exercise whether you are busy at work, with your family or if you have something else going on.

In addition, don't make excuses that you can't exercise because you are sick or tired or the weather is too cold or it is raining outside.

Instead do whatever it takes to get some exercise every day and that can be from running outside to doing some bodyweight exercises at home.

No matter what, have a fitness plan and be consistent with your training schedule.

Tip #25 Do Full Body Workouts

To make sure you burn the most amount of calories, focus on exercising your entire body by doing full body workouts.

Full body workouts are great because you will exercise the entire body in a short amount of time and burn a lot of calories.

Here are some circuit routines for a Full Body Workout:

<u>Circuit Routine 1 (4-6 Sets)</u>

- Bodyweight squats (12-15) repetitions
- Pushups (8-12) repetitions
- Sit-ups (10-15) repetitions
  *rest 1 minute

<u>Circuit Routine 2 (4-6 Sets)</u>

- Lunges (alternate forward and reverse) (12-15) repetitions
- Diamond Pushups (8-12) repetitions
- Bodyweight planks (30-45 seconds)
  *rest 1 minute

<u>**Circuit Routine 3 (4-6 Sets)**</u>

- Pushup Burpees (6-8) repetitions

- Flutter kicks (12-15) repetitions

- Mountain climbers (10-12) repetitions

  *rest 1 minute

Tip #26 Keep Track of Your Fitness Goals

Keep track of your health and fitness goals day after day, week after week, month after month.

You can do so by writing down your workouts and your progress. In addition, keep a food journal.

Try to write down what you ate and what time you ate especially if you are practicing the ketogenic diet or intermittent fasting or both.

Tip # 27 Prioritize Your Diet

Although exercise is great for the body, mind and spirit, when it comes to losing weight, it is all about your DIET.

Simply to be lean and stay in shape you really have to focus on your diet.

So, if you can really focus on your diet in addition to getting some daily exercise, you will be able to remain fit 365 days a year.

To make sure you are staying in shape day after day, week after week, month after month make every attempt to eat a lot of vegetables, nuts, lean meats and fruits.

You can also consider shopping at the local farmer's market to make sure that the food you are buying is fresh.

Tip #28 Do Some Exercise Early in The Morning

If you want to make sure you exercise every day, then simply try to go to sleep a little earlier so that you can wake up a little earlier to get a morning workout.

No matter how buys you may be, it is a good idea to wake up early and do some exercise immediately upon waking up.

Research shows that doing some form of light exercise upon waking up is a great way to get the body and mind ready for the day.

Your morning workout does not have to be long.

You can do a short, intense bodyweight circuit routine or you can simply go for a short 20-minute run or a 30-minute walk.

The point is you want to start your day by being active because later in the day you may get a little lazy and decide not to do any exercise especially if you feel tired.

Tip #29 Use A Standing Desk

A standing desk is a desk that is designed for a person to use while standing up.

A person can use a standing desk to comfortably read, write or do some work on a computer or laptop while standing up.

Research shows that you burn more calories when using a standing desk then when you sit down and use a traditional desk.

Simply, when you are standing up, your body is using more energy to remain standing versus when you sit down.

When you are sitting down at a traditional desk, all of your weight is being supported by a chair and many times that chair may not even be comfortable.

In addition, standing desks get you moving around more as well as walking around more because you are more motivated to walk or move around then if you sit down at a traditional desk which simply makes the body and mind too comfortable and lazy.

BONUS

Tip #30 Sleep Benefits for Weight Loss

Every busy person has a shortage of time. However, when it comes to sleep, a person must make time for getting enough sleep in order to succeed in overall life.

There are so many benefits to exercise and having a healthy diet. But when it truly comes to weight loss, sleep is the secret to fat loss.

Here are 8 reasons why sleep will help you to lose weight:

#1 Sleep Controls Your Diet and Fitness Lifestyle

Believe it or not but sleep is more important than diet and exercise.

The reason why sleep is more important than diet and exercise is because if you don't get enough sleep (7-9 hours) every night, your lack of sleep will negatively affect both your diet and your fitness goals.

Research shows that the more you sleep the more weight you lose because you will have the energy and focus to stick to your diet as well as to exercise with tremendous energy.

This concept of sleeping more to lose more weight is very simple yet very difficult to follow by many people especially busy people.

The solution is to make sleep a priority just like accomplishing your work, family and financial goals are a priority.

#2 Sleep Eliminates Food Cravings

Research shows that getting enough sleep eliminates food cravings because your body is not stressed from a lack of a good night's sleep.

However, when you don't get enough sleep, you cause your body to develop stress.

When you are stressed, this hormone called cortisol causes you to crave food especially unhealthy foods and what happens is that eventually you give in and begin to eat more and more.

Cortisol is responsible for weight gain so whenever your body produces cortisol, you will simply gain weight.

In order to prevent cortisol from developing in the body, you have to make sure you are getting enough sleep.

It does not matter how much you exercise or how strict your diet is. If you do not get enough sleep, your body will be craving food as a result of the stress it undergoes as a result of not getting enough sleep.

#3 Good Quality Sleep Builds Muscle

If you strength train and get a good night's sleep you allow your body to repair itself. In addition, you allow your body to build muscle as a result of getting a good night's sleep.

Building muscle is good for fighting fat because even if you have small amounts of muscle, this muscle will force your body to burn off calories.

#4 Sleep Is the Fountain of Youth

Whenever you get a good night's rest, your body develops Human Growth Hormone (HGH).

Human growth Hormone is a natural hormone that your body develops and is responsible for anti-aging.

More specifically, Human Growth Hormone enhances weight loss, develops stronger bones, builds muscle, reduces cardiovascular disease, improves your mood as well as your cognitive function.

Therefore, the more you sleep, the more Human Growth Hormone your body will develop.

As a result of developing more Human Growth Hormone, you will live longer and feel more youthful and energetic as a result of sleeping more.

#5 Sleep Gives You Superior Energy

When you get a good night of sleep, you wake up feeling refreshed ready to take on the world.

In addition, you will be more motivated to exercise, eat healthy and accomplish your daily goals as a result of getting a good night's sleep.

It is also important to state that getting a good night's sleep will give you razor sharp focus and a strong willingness to accomplish your daily goals.

#6 The More You Sleep the Less You Eat

Research shows that the earlier you go to sleep and the more you sleep (7-9 hours), the less likely you are to eat because you will be eliminating late night snacking and boredom from staying up late.

In addition, sleeping more will help to keep you focused on your diet and health and fitness lifestyle as a result of being well rested.

#7 Sleeping More Burns More Calories

Research shows that you burn more calories when you sleep between 7-9 hours per night then if you were to sleep between 4-6 hours per night.

The reason being is because when you sleep 7-9 hour per night, your body is working more efficiently at burning calories as a result of it being well rested.

However, if you only sleep between 4-6 hours per night, your body will be under tremendous stress and will feel lethargic making your body to burn less calories over time.

#8 A Good Night Sleep Will Help You to Shop for Healthy Foods

Research shows that people that get a good night's rest are likelier to eat healthier as well as shop for healthier food versus people that don't get enough sleep.

This is because people that don't get enough sleep tend to drink sugary drinks like coffee with extra sugar and energy drinks in order to stay awake.

In addition, a person that does not get a good night's rest will be stressed out and will be searching for comfort foods which most likely will be unhealthy foods.

Here are Some Tips for a Better Night's Sleep

- Turn off your computer, cell phone, and TV at least 30 minutes before you go to sleep.

- Make your bed and bedroom as relaxing as possible in order to ensure a good night's sleep.

- Create a nightly bedtime ritual. Consider taking a warm bath or reading a book before going to bed. In addition, eliminate doing any important work before going to bed.

- Develop a bedtime schedule. Figure out what time you want to wake up in the morning then decide to go to sleep every night at the same time making sure you sleep between 7-9 hours every night.

- Eliminate drinking any fluids before you go to sleep in order to prevent waking up at night to go to the toilet. In addition, eliminate drinking coffee early in the evening and stay away from energy drinks, soda and alcohol if possible.

- Try to sleep in complete darkness if possible. If this is uncomfortable consider buying a lamp with a timer that shuts off after a few minutes.

Summary

I hope you enjoyed the 30 of the Best Tips for Rapid Fat Loss.

To get the most out of this entire book, it is important for you to be persistent with achieving your health and fitness goals.

In addition, it is important to develop resilience and persevere when confronted with challenges along your health and fitness journey.

Learn to realize that every day, you should have a short list of your top three or four priorities in your life and exercise and living a health and fitness lifestyle should be one of them.

Nevertheless, take what you have learned from this book and apply it to your health and fitness lifestyle.

It can be stated that exercise and living a health and fitness lifestyle is one of the most important habits to have in life.

In addition, the power of exercise and living a health and fitness lifestyle can transform your body, mind and your overall life so embrace it with everything you got.

www.ingramcontent.com/pod-product-compliance
Lightning Source LLC
Chambersburg PA
CBHW070118260726
48658CB00001B/159